THE IBS COOKBOOK
COLLECTION

250 Low FODMAP Recipes

From The Essential IBS Cookbook and The IBS Slow Cooker Cookbook

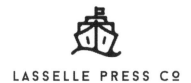

LASSELLE PRESS CO

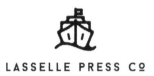

LASSELLE PRESS C⁰

ISBN-13: 978-1911364498
ISBN-10: 1911364499

CONTENTS

SEAFOOD | 61

POULTRY | 95

VEGETARIAN | 132

STOCKS, SOUPS AND STEWS | 164

SIDES, SALADS, SNACKS and SAUCES | 188

DRINKS AND DESSERTS | 208

SEAFOOD | 273

DRINKS AND DESSERTS | 284

CONVERSION TABLES | 292

BIBLIOGRAPHY | 294

INDEX | 295

INTRODUCTION

Welcome to The IBS Cookbook Collection!

We've put together this huge collection of 250 recipes from both The Essential IBS Cookbook and The IBS Slow Cooker Cookbook to provide you with delicious, easy to make low FODMAP meals. These meals have been put together to help manage and ease your symptoms of IBS.

Here at Lasselle Press, we understand that experiencing the symptoms of Irritable Bowel Syndrome (IBS) can be uncomfortable, painful and even embarrassing. If you've already been diagnosed then you will know that your lifestyle and diet will have to change. If you haven't been diagnosed but are experiencing uncomfortable symptoms, you are probably feeling confused, anxious and maybe even miserable. Either way, this book is aimed at helping you. You will need to seek a professional diagnosis before you make any changes to your diet and hopefully the information provided in the first part of this book will give you more insight and confidence to see your doctor or to speak to somebody about your symptoms. We go over what IBS is, its potential causes and symptoms, as well as providing information about the low FODMAP diet with extensive lists of foods you can continue to enjoy as well as those you should avoid. Cooking and lifestyle guidance is also given in order to make the transition to the low FODMAP diet the easiest and smoothest possible for you during this challenging time.

The rest of this book is dedicated to providing you with healthy and delicious recipes for breakfast, lunch, dinner and dessert that won't leave you feeling uninspired, worn out in the kitchen, or out of budget! We've added 50 slow cooker recipes for when time is of the essence, so that you can get on with life without the stress and hassle of working out what to eat and spending hours in the kitchen. Each recipe contains easy-to-find ingredients, simple instructions and tastes amazing! Each recipe is also given with its nutritional value broken down, to help you plan your meals and keep track of what you're eating. Hopefully this will take the strain out of meal planning and preparation, and allow you and the family to enjoy dinner time again.

We wish you all the best in the kitchen and in health!

The Lasselle Press Team

C1: IBS OVERVIEW

IBS affects the large intestine and can cause changes and discomfort during bowel movements. These range in severity from person to person and can be inconvenient, uncomfortable and sometimes even debilitating. Unfortunately the syndrome is incurable, but it can be managed with long term treatment, diet and lifestyle choices.

The exact cause of IBS is unknown, however it may be caused by a problem in the interaction between the gut, the brain and the nervous system. Some factors, such as stress, can worsen symptoms of IBS whilst they do not cause it. Surprisingly very few people seek medical help despite suffering from the symptoms of IBS; in the US, most patients finally seek help around six years after the symptoms of IBS start. It is essential that you do seek a professional diagnosis of IBS if you are concerned that you may be experiencing the symptoms of the syndrome, or if you have a family history of IBS.

According to www.aboutibs.org, 'IBS affects between 25 and 45 million people in the United States.' Of these, two thirds are female. IBS can affect people of all age ranges but is most prevalent in those under 50 years old and can also affect children. Unfortunately it is a syndrome that many are embarrassed to get help for or talk about with their peers due to the nature of the syndrome's symptoms. Thus many end up worsening their symptoms through not getting suitable help and guidance. Treatments are available to help manage IBS and as previously mentioned, changes in your diet and lifestyle can help lessen symptoms which vary from person to person.

So don't lose hope if you've recently been diagnosed, or think you might be suffering from IBS. Seek medical opinion, talk to a trusted family member or friend, and know that there are things that can be changed in order to relieve the pain and discomfort you may be currently feeling.

Symptoms of IBS

There are a variety of symptoms associated with IBS and these can often coincide. These include:
- Diarrhoea
- Constipation
- Abdominal pain and cramping
- Gas
- Feeling bloated
- Mucus in the stool

You should seek out medical help if you develop symptoms of rectal bleeding, abdominal pain that becomes severely worse at night, or unexplained weight loss. These are symptoms that could worsen the overall effects of IBS, or could point to more serious underlying issues with your health.

There are two categories of IBS:

IBS-D - resulting in diarrhoea symptoms.

IBS-C - resulting in constipation symptoms.

Although there are two categories, it is important to remember that your symptoms can alternate and shift between the two.

IBS Triggers

Although as previously mentioned, the exact cause of IBS is unknown, we know how it occurs in comparison to a healthy intestinal tract system in a person without IBS: layers of muscle line the walls of our intestines that either contract or relax in order to move the food we consume from our stomach all the way down to our rectum, through the intestinal tract. With IBS, these contractions may either be stronger, lasting longer than usual, thus causing gas, bloating, and diarrhoea, or they may be weaker and slower than usual, thus causing constipation.
There are many different triggers for the symptoms of IBS to occur; these range from person to person, and can also change over time for a particular individual. It is important to keep all possible triggers in mind because of IBS being a terribly unpredictable syndrome. Some of the most common triggers are:

- Specific foods - this can vary between individuals.
  Food allergies or intolerances e.g. chocolate, spices, fat, beans, fruits, cauliflower, cabbage, broccoli, milk, soda, carbonated drinks, alcohol etc.
- Stress - triggers an over-active nervous system which can intensify the signals sent to the gastrointestinal area of the body and cause stronger contractions.
- Hormones - particularly worsening during a woman's menstrual cycle.
- Other illnesses e.g. anxiety or depression.
  Excess intestinal bacteria - can interfere with the digestion process and contribute to IBS symptoms.

Other Conditions Linked To IBS

What makes diagnosing and treating IBS a little complicated is that there are other conditions and diseases which are linked to the syndrome. These can produce similar symptoms and in some cases worsen IBS symptoms. Please discuss these conditions and symptoms with your doctor in order to receive suitable and specific treatment.

SIBO - a condition linked to and associated with IBS. SIBO stands for Small Intestine Bacteria Overgrowth. This overgrowth can interfere with the digestion process and absorption of food as well as damage the membrane lining. It is healthy to have a certain amount of bacteria in our gut. In this case however, there will be an excessive amount of bacteria; this can cause chronic fatigue, body pains, and stress on the liver. Through the damage caused to the membrane lining, larger food particles are able to pass through without being properly digested; this can cause food allergies and sensitivities. If you are diagnosed and treated for SIBO, your IBS symptoms may also be alleviated.

Celiac Disease - another condition linked to IBS. Celiac Disease causes a sensitivity to gluten. Gluten is a protein that is contained in barley, rye, and wheat products. Celiac disease can cause symptoms such as anemia, fatigue, diarrhoea, bloating and weight loss, which can sometimes lead to serious complications. Celiac disease can worsen IBS symptoms.

In the next chapter we will discuss dietary and lifestyle changes you can make in order to help relieve the symptoms of IBS.

C2: DIET AND LIFESTYLE GUIDANCE

Along with the treatment prescribed by your doctor and their guidance, making changes to your diet and lifestyle can have an extremely positive effect on your symptoms and your lifestyle. There are a number of different diets that have been recommended for IBS sufferers and each person will react differently to certain foods, so it is important to bear this in mind. Be mindful of which foods trigger your symptoms as well as those that do not; you can do this by keeping a journal of the foods and drinks you eat as well as your symptoms experienced daily. This method will allow you to notice if there are any patterns with certain foods or ingredients that may be triggering symptoms.

This cookbook uses low FODMAP foods as the diet that is most commonly now recommended for those with IBS. Again, this may vary from patient to patient and it is imperative to seek dietary guidance from a professional before changing your diet. Information about the low FODMAP diet will be given in the next section so that you can find out more about it.

The Low FODMAP Diet

FODMAPs stand for Fermentable, Oligio-, Di-, Mono-saccharides And Polyols. FODMAPs are carbohydrates with short chains that naturally occur in food and are not properly absorbed through the small intestine. Choosing foods and portion sizes that are low in FODMAPs can greatly reduce the triggering of symptoms.

- Use the lists on the following pages to select foods and portion sizes that are classed as Low FODMAP.
- Avoid those that are classed as high FODMAP.

Please note, whilst some foods may be classed as low FODMAP, this can depend on the portion size. Take note of the portion sizes for each type of food and ingredient so that you don't go over the recommended serving sizes.

Fruits:
LOW FODMAP - Enjoy (stick to 1 fruit/1 cup per serving whichever is the smaller quantity):
Banana (1/2 large banana serving/approx. 30g),
Blueberries – buy organic,
Boysenberry – buy organic,
Cantaloupe,
Star fruit,
Cranberry – buy organic,
Grapes – buy organic,
Grapefruit,
Honeydew melon,
Kiwi,
Lemon,
Lime,
Mandarin,
Orange,
Passion fruit,
Paw paw,
Pineapple,
Raspberry – buy organic,
Rhubarb,
Strawberry – buy organic,
Tangelo.

HIGH FODMAP - Avoid - (any fruits of more than 1 cup per serving) plus:
Apple,
Mango,
Nashi fruit,
Pear,
Persimmon,
Watermelon,
Persimmon,
Rambutan,
Apricot,
Avocado,
Blackberries,
Cherries,

Longon,
Lychee,
Nectarine,
Peach,
Plum,
Prunes.

VEGETABLES: Enjoy (stick to 1 vegetable/1 cup per serving whichever is the smaller quantity):
Alfalfa,
Bamboo Shoots,
Bean Shoots,
Beans (Green),
Bok Choy,
Capsicum,
Carrot (1 Medium Carrot),
Celery,
Chives (Green Section Only),
Choy Sum,
Cucumber,
Endive,
Fennel Heart (1 Small Heart Or Smaller 49G),
Ginger,
Lettuce (May Be Okay For Some),
Marrow,
Olives,
Parsnip,
Parsley,
Potato (2 Small Potatoes),
Pumpkin (1/2 Cup),
Silver Beet,
Scallion (Green Section Only),
Spinach (1 Cup),
Swede,
Sweet Potato (3 Tbsp),
Taro,
Beef Tomatoes,
Turnip,

Yam,
Eggplant,
Zucchini (this may be okay for some; check individual tolerance).

Avoid (any vegetables of more than 1 cup per serving) plus:
Artichokes (Globe And Jerusalem),
Asparagus,
Beets,
Broccoli,
Brussel Sprouts,
Cabbage,
Chicory,
Dandelion Leaves,
Garlic,
Legumes, Okra, Onion (Brown, White, And Spanish), Peas, Radicchio Lettuce, Shallots, Leeks, Scallions And Chives (White Sections),
Squash ,
Cauliflower,
Mushrooms,
Snow Peas And Sugar Snap Peas,
Corn,
Cherry Tomatoes (due to mould).
Please note: there is undeclared onion hidden in many processed foods including, chicken salt, vegetable salt, vegetable powder, dehydrated vegetables, stocks, gravies, soups, marinades, and sauces. Make sure you check ingredients labels for packaged items and avoid onion.

Flavorings and Herbs and Spices
Enjoy:
Pecans (Max 15 Per Serving), Walnuts,
Golden Syrup, Treacle, Molasses, Maple Syrup,
White, Brown, Raw And Castor Sugar, (Sucrose) Eaten In Moderation,
Tea And Herbal Teas,
Seeds (In Moderation),
Oat Bran (Max 1/4 Cup Serving), Rolled Oats (Max 1/4 Cup Serving), Gluten Free Oats,
Barley Bran, Psyllium, Rice Bran,
Stevia, Baking Cocoa Powder, Carob Powder,
Olive Oil, Canola Oil, Garlic-Infused Oil, Coconut Oil,

Unsweetened Desiccated Coconut (Max 1/4 Cup Serving),
Fresh And Dried Ginger, Cilantro, Basil, Lemongrass, Mint, Parsley, Marjoram, Thyme,
Rosemary And Other Herbs.

Avoid:
Honey, Corn Syrups, Fruisana,
Chicory And Dandelion Tea,
Artificial Sweeteners,
Sugar Free Or Low Carb Sweets, Mints Or Gums,
Dairy Desserts,
Baked Beans, Lentils, Chickpeas,
Solid Chocolate, Solid Carob, Olives,
Nuts And Nut Butters,
Caffeine, Decaf Coffee.

Dairy and Other
Enjoy:
Egg Whites,
Rice Milk, Almond Milk, Raw Goats Milk, Hemp Milk,
Goats Cheese, Cottage Cheese.

Avoid:
Other Cheeses,
Egg Yolks,
Dairy (Milk, Cream, Yogurt, Butter, Sour Cream),
Soy Milk, Coconut Milk,
Vegetable Oils.

Wheat Products and Alternatives:
Enjoy:
Rice, Amaranth, Tapioca, Quinoa, Millet, Sorghum, Buckwheat, Arrowroot, Sago,
Gluten Free (GF) Bread, Gluten Free Pasta,
Rice Noodles, Wheat Free Buckwheat Noodles,
Porridge, Wheat Free Muesli, Rice Bubbles, Gluten Free Cereals, Rice Cakes And
Crackers, GF Crackers, Ryvitas, GF Cakes, Flourless Cakes, GF Biscuits, GF Pastry
Mixes And Bread Crumbs,
Polenta, Buckwheat, Millet And Rice Flours.

Avoid:
Bread (white, wholemeal, multigrain, sourdough, pita, and many rye),
Pasta and Noodles (regular, two minute, spelt, egg noodles, hokkien and udon),
Breakfast Cereals (containing wheat, excess dried fruit and/or fruit juice),
Savory Biscuits (wheat based),
Cakes and Baked Goods (wheat based), Biscuits (wheat based),
Pastry and Breadcrumbs (wheat flour made),
Others (semolina, couscous, bulgur).

Protein Sources:
Enjoy:
Oily Fish,
Lean Meats e.g. Skinless Chicken or Turkey Breasts.

Avoid:
Red Meat,
Dark Meat From Poultry e.g. Turkey/Chicken Thighs,
Soy Products e.g. Tofu/Tempeh.

Lifestyle Guidance

Along with a diet that prevents or lessens the trigger of your IBS symptoms, other lifestyle changes can help you to feel healthier and less stressed, thus alleviating symptoms further.

1.   Ensure you exercise regularly - 20-30 minutes per day or 2-3 times per week will boost serotonin levels, helping you to feel happier and less stressed. Additionally you will feel great physically and prevent other serious illnesses such as obesity and heart disease.

2.   Eat your meals slowly and mindfully. In other words, not at your computer on a 'working lunch', rushing to pick up the kids, or on the way to work. This will help to prevent the symptoms such as cramps and bloating.

3.   Avoid chewing gum, especially when you're not eating soon after. The saliva that builds in your mouth sends a signal to your stomach that you are about to eat, if this is not the case it confuses the digestive system and can trigger symptoms.

4.   Drink plenty of water! This greatly improves general health as well as assisting the digestive system in flushing out slow to move particles and preventing constipation.

5.   Evaluate your work/life balance. Is the commute causing you unnecessary stress? Is there someone who can possibly help with the childcare or chores in any way? Can you cut down on unnecessary expenses so that you have more money to pay for childcare? Whatever helps prevent or cut down stress can have a dramatic positive effect on your symptoms.

6.   Try to get plenty of sleep by winding down at least one hour before you would like to be asleep and turning off all computers and electronic devices. Use an alarm clock rather than your phone and turn off anything electric at the wall; the blue lighting and signals can interfere with your brain waves and keep you alert when you want to be fast asleep!

7.   IBS can be a source of embarrassment to many sufferers and many end up concealing their symptoms or avoiding situations because of them. IBS can really affect the way you get on with everyday life. Reach out to a local support group or to online forums if you don't want to discuss it with family and friends. Talk to your doctors for advice. If you can, tell someone at work who you feel you can trust so that you don't find yourself having to make up excuses for sick days or even mid shift. You will be surprised at how understanding your colleagues and employers can be!

8.   Consider therapies - counselling can be extremely helpful; as with any other physical or mental illness, IBS can cause mental and physical symptoms. Consider cognitive behavioural therapy, hypnotherapy, biofeedback and others. Your local support group, doctors or the internet may be able to help you work out what type of therapy would benefit you the most.

9.   Take a look at your medications - some medications prescribed to you may actually be worsening the symptoms of IBS including: antibiotics, some antidepressants, and medicine containing sorbitol such as cough syrups, prozac, sarafem and zoloft can cause diarrhoea. Speak to your doctor about any current medication you're on and whether they these can be adjusted to your needs. Always consult your doctor before discontinuing any medications.

C3: EATING OUT AND TRAVEL GUIDE

Advice for Dining Out

It can be very hard for you to dine out with friends and family if you suffer from IBS; you never know when your symptoms might be triggered and what foods may or may not be available. But you don't have to miss out on your favorite restaurant or cuisines! Here are a few tips that may make dining out easier for you:

- Research the restaurant's menu beforehand and decide what you will choose to avoid anxiety and spontaneous decisions on the night.
- Use the food lists in the previous chapter to help you choose and don't feel bad about asking the restaurant to cater to your needs.
- Ask your server for your foods to be cooked without extra salts, butters or sauces.
- Avoid fried foods and opt for grilled or poached instead.
- Avoid drinking alcohol and opt for water or lemonade instead.
- Eat slowly and pace yourself between courses.
- Take any medication you have been prescribed at the usual time.

Advice for traveling

1. Whatever your travel plans, you will have to eat. If you plan ahead, you should be able to make a meal plan that suits your need.
2. If you have a dietitian, tell them where you are going and what you expect to eat at your destination.
3. Remember to pack enough of any prescription medicines you must take.
4. If going on a road trip or camping, avoid processed meats and foods.
5. Take snacks suitable for the low FODMAP diet to avoid picking up treats from the service stations!
6. Do not consume dairy products.
7. If you are going on a cruise, all those buffet foods are tempting to eat 24 hours a day. To help with this predicament try to select fruits, salads, and vegetables from the low FODMAP lists.
8. Let the cruise line or hotel know of your dietary needs, most are willing to prepare special foods for you.
9. If you are going to be traveling abroad and don't speak the language, take a phrasebook that has a section for ordering food.
10. Check if you can check in early and check out late to avoid waiting around for flight times.

Cooking Tips

1. *Grill, poach, roast or sauté meats instead of frying.*
2. *Steam or boil vegetables instead of frying.*
3. *Use healthy oils such as extra virgin olive oil or coconut oil to shallow fry.*
4. *Avoid added sugars and opt for Stevia instead of sugar.*
5. *Herbs are more likely to calm the digestive system and your gut while spices are more likely to irritate it. Oregano, basil, parsley, sage, mint, thyme, cilantro, ginger, and cloves are great herbs to incorporate into your meals. You want to avoid spices like cayenne pepper, chili powder or any hot sauces.*

Useful Kitchen Equipment

*   A selection of non-stick skillets,
*   A large pot for soups and stews,
*   A Slow Cooker,
*   A set of Tupperware for storage and bulk cooking,
*   Food Processor/blender/mortar and pestle
*   Large Bowls for salads or mixing.

One Last Thing

Always remember to use new recipes and ingredients after speaking to your doctor or dietitian; your needs will be unique to you depending on your symptoms and the certain foods that trigger them.
We hope that with your doctor's advice, along with our guidance and recipes, that you can continue to enjoy cooking, eating and sharing meal times with your loved ones.

Thank you for purchasing this book and we wish you all the best on your path to health and contentment.

Happy cooking!

BREAKFAST

Strawberry Oats

SERVES 1 / PREP TIME: 5 MINUTES / COOK TIME: 15 MINUTES

Delicious pops of sweetness combine with the crunch of the muesli in this simple breakfast recipe.

2 tbsp wheat-free muesli for topping (optional)
1 tsp maple syrup
¼ cup rolled oats (or gluten-free if celiac)
½ cup almond milk

1/4 cup organic strawberries, sliced

1. Preheat the oven to its highest setting.
2. To make the muesli -combine the maple syrup with the muesli and layer across a lined baking tray.
3. Place in the oven for 10 minutes or until crunchy.
4. Combine the oats and milk and cook in a pan over low heat for 3-4 minutes or according to package directions (alternatively pop this in the microwave for 1 minute).
5. Serve and scatter with strawberries and the crunchy muesli topping.

Hint: Make extra crunchy muesli and store in an airtight container for up to 2 weeks. It makes a great addition to any breakfast.

Per serving: Calories: 417 Protein: 11g Carbs: 79g Fiber: 9g Sugar: 24g Fat: 7g

Banana and Cocoa Oatmeal Pancakes

SERVES 2 / PREP TIME: 10 MINUTES / COOK TIME: 5 MINUTES

Filling and sweet – great for breakfast and dessert!

---

2 large egg whites
1 ½ cup rolled oats (gluten-free if celiac)
½ cup almond milk
1 medium banana
1 tsp vanilla extract
2 tbsp baking cocoa powder

2 tsp coconut oil

---

1. First, blend together the egg whites, oats, almond milk, banana and vanilla extract in a food processor until you get a smooth mixture.
2. Pour your mixture into a medium sized bowl and then add the cocoa powder.
3. Heat 1 tsp the oil in a large skillet on medium heat.
4. Once the oil is hot, pour half of your pancake batter into the skillet and leave for 4-5 minutes.
5. Use a spatula to gently place under the edges of the pancake – if it comes away from the skillet easily then flip the pancake over and continue to cook for 2-3 minutes.
6. Lower the heat if needed to prevent burning.
7. Repeat for the second pancake.
8. Top with a little maple syrup if desired.

Hint: You could try swapping the oats for the same amount of rice milk and make banana crépes instead.

Per serving: Calories: 360 Protein: 14g Carbs: 62g Fiber: 10g Sugar: 12g Fat: 8g

Homemade Granola

SERVES 2 / PREP TIME: 5 MINUTES / COOK TIME: 40 MINUTES

It can be extremely difficult to find cereals when you're suffering with IBS; the good news is that it is so simple to make!

---

1 cup rolled oats (gluten-free if need-ed)
1 tbsp uncooked quinoa
1 tbsp flax seeds
1 cup organic raspberries
Zest of 1 orange
1 tbsp maple syrup
1 tsp stevia powder

1 tbsp coconut oil (melted)

---

1. Preheat the oven to 300°F/ 150°C/Gas Mark 2.
2. Mix the oats, quinoa, flax seeds, raspberries and orange zest in a large bowl.
3. Add the maple syrup, stevia and oil and stir until combined.
4. Layer the mixture across a lined baking tray.
5. Bake in the oven for 35-40 minutes, mixing occasionally with a wooden spoon.
6. The granola should be golden brown and smelling delicious by now!
7. Remove from the oven and allow to cool before serving.
8. Enjoy on its own or with your choice of dairy-free milk.

Hint: This can be stored in an airtight container for up to three days in the refrigerator, so go ahead and make in bulk to save time! You can also substitute raspberries for any LOW FODMAP fruit of your choice. Skip the fruit to store for 2-3 weeks and simply add fresh fruit to serve.

Per serving: Calories: 333 Protein: 8g Carbs: 51g Fiber: 10g Sugar: 10g Fat: 12g

Spinach and Goats Cheese Frittata

SERVES 5 / PREP TIME: 10 MINUTES / COOK TIME: 25 MINUTES

A tasty start to the day!

---

2 small white potatoes, peeled and sliced
1 tsp olive oil
4 cups baby spinach
1 tsp canola oil
5 egg whites
½ cup goats cheese
1 tbsp parsley (dried or fresh)
A pinch of salt and pepper to taste

---

1. Add the sliced potatoes to a pan of boiling water over high heat and boil for 7-8 minutes.
2. Meanwhile, heat the olive oil in a non-stick skillet over medium heat.
3. Next, add the baby spinach to the skillet and cook for 5 minutes or until wilted.
4. Drain any excess water from the skillet and place spinach to one side.
5. Now drain the potatoes and allow to cool slightly.
6. Reheat the skillet and add the canola oil.
7. Sauté the potato slices for 5-6 minutes or until golden.
8. Preheat your broiler/grill on high and whisk together the egg whites, goats cheese, spinach, parsley and salt and pepper.
9. Pour the egg mixture into the skillet with the potatoes.
10. Place under the broiler/grill for 10 minutes until eggs are thoroughly cooked through and the top is golden and bubbling.
11. Slice into five portions and enjoy!

Per serving: Calories: 120 Protein: 9g Carbs: 8g Fiber: 2g Sugar: 1g Fat: 6g

Buckwheat Porridge with Grapefruit

SERVES 2 / PREP TIME: 5 MINUTES / COOK TIME: 25 MINUTES

Buckwheat is a Low FODMAP alternative for breakfast and tastes amazing.

---

1 cup buckwheat groats
2 cups rice/almond/hemp milk
1 cup fresh grapefruit, sliced
2 tsp stevia

---

1. Over medium heat, combine the buckwheat and milk in a pot and bring to a simmer.
2. Cook with the lid on for 18-20 minutes.
3. The buckwheat will have soaked up most of the milk once done.
4. Remove and serve with the sliced grapefruit and a sprinkle of stevia powder to counteract the sour taste of the grapefruit.

Per serving: Calories: 361 Protein: 10g Carbs: 76g Fiber: 9g Sugar: 26g Fat: 4g

Low-Carb Chia Pumpkin Flapjacks

SERVES 4 / PREP TIME: 10 MINUTES / COOK TIME: 10 MINUTES

These hearty oat, chia, and pumpkin flapjacks will start your day off right!

1 tbsp chia seeds
1 tbsp golden flax seed meal
2 tbsp maple syrup
1/4 cup unsweetened almond/rice milk
A pinch of salt
1/2 tsp pumpkin pie spice
1/2 cup canned pumpkin purée

1/4 cup rice flour
Olive oil cooking spray
Maple syrup to taste

1. In a medium sized bowl, combine the chia seeds, the golden flax seed meal, the syrup, and the milk.
2. Let this mixture sit for 5 minutes.
3. Next, fold in the salt, the pumpkin pie spice, the pumpkin purée, and the rice flour.
4. Mix everything in the bowl thoroughly.
5. Meanwhile, heat your pan or griddle to medium heat.
6. Spray with olive oil cooking spray.
7. Now pour the flapjack mixture into the pan or griddle in four evenly sized circles.
8. Spread each circle with a spatula until it reaches about 2-3 inches in diameter.
9. Cook over medium heat for 4-5 minutes.
10. Flip the flapjacks over and cook for the same amount of time.
11. Serve hot.

Hint: Use a non-stick frying pan or griddle to prevent the flapjacks from sticking.

Per serving: Calories: 108   Protein: 2g Carbs: 20g Sugar: 9g Fat: 2g

Sunrise Pancakes

SERVES 4 / PREP TIME: 10 MINUTES / COOK TIME: 10 MINUTES

This delightful combination of sesame seeds and banana is sure to power up your morning!

---

1 tbsp sesame seeds
1/4 cup steel cut oats (gluten-free)
1 medium ripe banana
1 egg white
1/2 tsp ground ginger
1 tbsp coconut flakes
Olive oil cooking spray

---

1. In a clean spice or coffee grinder, blend the sesame seeds and oats until the combination has a flour-like texture.
2. In a separate small food processor, blend together the banana, the egg white, and the ginger until it the mixture is smooth.
3. Pour the oat and sesame flour into the banana batter and blend in the food processor again until all is thoroughly combined.
4. After blending, take the food processor bowl off and mix in the coconut flakes with a spoon.
5. Set aside the batter so it can thicken.
6. While the batter thickens, preheat your frying pan or griddle and spray with olive oil cooking spray.
7. Divide the batter into four pancakes in the pan.
8. Spread out each pancake with a spatula to about 3 inches in diameter.
9. Cook the pancakes over medium heat for 4-5 minutes on the first side.
10. Flip them with a spatula and cook them about 3-4 minutes on the second side, until they are golden brown.
11. Serve.

Tip: Instead of using a food processor, you can mash the ripe banana with a fork and briskly whisk the egg white and cinnamon through until the mixture is smooth.

Per serving: Calories: 99 Protein: 2g Carbs: 12g Fiber: 2g Sugar: 4g Fat: 2g

Hearty Homemade Energy Bars

SERVES 8 / PREP TIME: 10 MINUTES / COOK TIME: 30 MINUTES

These easy energy bars are sure to make snack time fun and healthy.

3/4 cup oat flour
1/4 cup unsweetened coconut flakes
1/2 tsp baking powder
1 ripe banana, mashed
1/4 cup maple syrup

1/2 tsp vanilla extract
1/4 cup dry roasted pumpkin seeds
1/4 cup dry roasted sunflower seeds, hulled
1/8 cup chia seeds

1. Preheat the oven to 350 degrees.
2. Line an 8x8 oven-safe dish with parchment paper.
3. Combine the oat flour, the coconut flakes, the baking powder, the mashed banana, the maple syrup, and the vanilla extract in a large bowl and mix thoroughly.
4. Stir in the pumpkin seeds, the sunflower seeds, and the chia seeds.
5. Mix everything together until well combined.
6. Scrape the mixture into the lined baking dish and level it out with wet fingers.
7. Bake for 20 minutes at 350 degrees.
8. Turn the oven off.
9. Allow the mixture to sit in the warm oven for 5-10 minutes.
10. Remove the dish and allow it to cool on a wire rack.
11. Once it has cooled, turn the baked mixture onto a cutting board.
12. Slice into 8 bars and serve!

Per serving: Calories: 177 Protein: 5g Carbs: 26g Sugar: 9g Fat: 7g

Kiwi Chia Parfait

SERVES 6 / PREP TIME: 10 MINUTES / COOK TIME: NA / CHILL: OVERNIGHT

This breakfast treat is ready as soon as you wake up!

1/4 cup chia seeds
1/4 cup unsweetened coconut flakes
1 1/4 cup unsweetened light coconut milk
2 tbsp maple syrup
1 medium banana, mashed
3 kiwis, peeled and sliced

1 dash vanilla extract
A pinch of salt

---

1. Combine the chia seeds and the coconut in a large bowl.
2. Pour in the rest of the ingredients.
3. Stir everything in the bowl thoroughly, making sure the banana is smoothly incorporated.
4. Arrange the kiwi slices in alternating layers with the chia mixture in 6 sundae glasses or parfait bowls.
5. Cover with plastic wrap or aluminum foil.
6. Place in the refrigerator overnight.
7. Take out a spoon and enjoy first thing!

Hint: If you don't have sundae glasses or parfait bowls, just use pint-sized mason jars or glasses!

Per serving: Calories: 149 Protein: 3g Carbs: 11g Sugar: 10g Fat: 8g

Tomato and Chive Frittata

SERVES 2 / PREP TIME: 10 MINUTES / COOK TIME: 20 MINUTES

This Mediterranean-style breakfast will start your day right!

---

4 egg whites
6 tbsp unsweetened rice milk or water
A pinch of salt
1/2 cup fresh spinach, loosely chopped

1/2 fresh red bell pepper, diced
1/2 cup fresh roma tomatoes, diced
1/4 cup crumbled goat cheese
2 tbsp chives (green tips only), sliced

---

1. Whisk the egg whites in a large bowl until frothy.
2. Add in the milk and the salt.
3. Whisk these together until thoroughly combined.
4. Mix in the rest of the ingredients and stir well.
5. Meanwhile, preheat the oven to 350 degrees.
6. Place an oven-safe frying pan with a matching lid on the stovetop over medium heat.
7. Once the pan is warm, pour in the egg mixture.
8. Cover with the lid.
9. Let this pan sit over medium heat without stirring for about 5 minutes.
10. Next, place the pan in the oven.
11. Let it bake for 10-15 minutes.
12. Keep checking to see if the frittata is done. It is cooked when the top is no longer runny.
13. Remove from the oven.
14. Take off the lid and allow it to cool for a couple of minutes before serving.

Per serving: Calories: 236 Protein: 18g Carbs: 16g Sugar: 12g Fat: 12g

Vegetarian Miso Pasta To Go

SERVES 2 / PREP TIME: 10 MINUTES / COOK TIME: 2 MINUTES

This jarred dinner can be made ahead of time and grabbed for an on-the-go meal.

1/2 tsp miso paste
1/4 tsp onion infused olive oil
1/4 tsp garlic-infused olive oil
1/2 cup chopped Swiss chard
1/4 cup finely grated carrot
4 tbsp rinsed canned sweet corn

1 (8 oz) bags rice vermicelli noodles (or equivalent gluten free noodle)
1 tbsp fresh chopped cilantro leaves
1 tbsp fresh minced scallions, green tips
2 wedges lemon
3-4 cups boiling water

---

1. Gather two 2 ¼ cup-capacity glass jars that are heatproof and can be sealed.
2. In a small bowl, mix together the miso paste and infused oils, then spread this mixture over the bottom of each jar.
3. Layer the rest of the ingredients equally in each jar as follows: the Swiss chard, the grated carrot, the sweet corn, the vermicelli noodles, the cilantro leaves, the scallions, and a wedge of lemon.
4. Pour 1 ½ - 2 cups boiling water over the contents of each jar.
5. Let the noodles cook in the water for 2 minutes before enjoying.

Hint: You can infuse your own olive oil by adding dried herbs to a jar of olive oil, sealing, storing it for a week, then straining.

Per serving: Calories: 138 Protein: 3 Carbs: 27 Sugar: 2 Fat: 2

Strawberry Chocolate Chia Pudding

SERVES 2 / PREP TIME: 5 MINUTES / COOK TIME: NA CHILL TIME: OVERNIGHT

A winning combination gives you something to look forward to when you wake up!

---

1 cup unsweetened almond/rice milk
1 ½ tsp maple syrup
1 tsp vanilla extract
1 tbsp unsweetened cocoa powder
2 tbsp chia seeds
1 cup fresh strawberries, sliced
2 tbsp unsweetened coconut flakes

---

1. Whisk the milk, maple syrup, vanilla extract, and cocoa powder together in a bowl.
2. Keep whisking until thoroughly mixed.
3. Stir in the chia seeds.
4. Pour into a glass jar.
5. Tightly cover with a lid.
6. Refrigerate overnight.
7. Just before serving, stir the pudding well to break up any lumps.
8. Pour the pudding into 2 serving bowls.
9. Scatter the sliced strawberries and the coconut flakes on top.
10. Store this pudding for up to 5 days in the fridge.

Hint: Add other low FODMAP toppings of your choice to mix this breakfast up.

Per serving: Calories: 149 Protein: 5g Carbs: 19g Sugar: 8g Fat: 7g

Homemade Millet Hot Cereal

SERVES 4 / PREP TIME: 5 MINUTES / COOK TIME: 25 MINUTES

This warming porridge fits perfectly in any balanced diet.

---

1 cup hulled millet seeds
1 cup unsweetened light coconut milk
1 ½ cups boiling water
Pinch of salt

Topping choices:
1 ripe banana
2 cups raspberries
1/2 cup pineapple chunks
1 tbsp maple syrup

---

1. Toast the millet seeds in a saucepan over a medium high heat for about 2-3 minutes, or until they start to turn golden.
2. Add the milk, boiling water, and salt.
3. Cover and bring to a simmer.
4. Once boiling, turn down the heat to the lowest setting.
5. Allow the pan to simmer for 15 to 20 minutes, or until most of the liquid absorbs and the millet is soft.
6. Turn off the burner.
7. After it's done cooking, stir more milk into the millet until the porridge is creamy.
8. Meanwhile, peel and slice the banana.
9. Gather the raspberries and pineapple chunks.
10. Divide the porridge among 4 bowls.
11. Top each bowl with the banana, raspberries, and pineapple slices.
12. Drizzle maple syrup over the fruit and serve.

Tip: You can include any other low FODMAP topping you like on top of this hot cereal, such as blueberries, strawberries, and so on.

Per serving: Calories: 375 Protein: 8 Carbs: 67 Sugar: 15 Fat: 11

Fresh Zucchini-Carrot Mini Frittatas

SERVES 5-6 / PREP TIME: 15 MINUTES / COOK TIME: 30 MINUTES

These muffin-sized frittatas are great to make ahead of time and eat for breakfast all week

---

2 large carrots, peeled and diced
1/4 cup olive oil
4 large egg whites
1 1/4 cups almond/rice milk
2 tsp garlic-infused olive oil
1/2 tsp ground turmeric

3/4 cup gluten-free all purpose baking flour
1 cup diced scallions (green tips)
1/3 cup fresh cilantro leaves, chopped
1 cup zucchini, grated
1 cup canned chickpeas, drained and rinsed
A pinch of salt and pepper to taste

---

1. Preheat the oven to 350 degrees.
2. Place a large frying pan over medium heat.
3. Meanwhile, peel and dice the carrots.
4. Add the carrots to the pan with a drizzle of the olive oil.
5. Allow the carrots to gently sauté for 10 to 15 minutes, or until soft and slightly golden brown, stirring occasionally.
6. Whisk together in a large bowl the egg whites, milk, and garlic infused oil.
7. Next, sprinkle in the turmeric and the flour, whisking until combined.
8. Mix the grated scallions, cilantro, zucchini, chickpeas, and cooked carrot into the bowl with the egg white mixture.
9. Season this mixture with salt and pepper to taste, then mix again.
10. Meanwhile, line one 12-muffin tin with muffin papers.
11. Spoon the frittata batter into each muffin cup, filling each cup almost to the top.
12. Place the muffin tin in the oven and cook for 25 to 30 minutes.
13. They are done when each mini frittata is springy and golden, or a skewer comes out clean.

Hint: It's normal for the frittatas to sink a little after coming out of the oven.

Tip: These will keep in the fridge for two days.

Per serving: Calories: 286 Protein: 9g Carbs: 33g Sugar: 8g Fat: 14g

Blueberries and Cream Rice Pudding

SERVES 4 / PREP TIME: 5 MINUTES / COOK TIME: 1 1/2 HOURS

If you like rice pudding, this blueberry variation will really satisfy your taste buds.

1/2 cup short grain white rice
1 1/2 tbsp chia seeds
2 cups canned light coconut milk
3 cups hemp milk
1/4 cup water

1/2 tsp ground ginger
Maple syrup to taste
2 cups organic blueberries
1/3 cup water

1. Preheat the oven to 320 degrees.
2. Place the rice, chia seeds, coconut milk, hemp milk, water, and ginger in a 9x13 baking dish.
3. Mix well.
4. Place the dish in the oven, uncovered.
5. Cook for 1 ½ hours, stirring every 20 to 30 minutes to break up the skin that forms on top.
6. While the rice is in the oven, place the blueberries into a small saucepan.
7. Add the 1/3 cup water to the blueberries and cover the pan with a lid.
8. Place it over medium heat for 5-6 minutes, or until the fruit is soft.
9. Remove the rice dish once the rice is thick and creamy like rice pudding.
10. Place the rice pudding to one side and it allow to cool for a few minutes.
11. Check the pudding to see if it has cooled down.
12. Stir in the blueberries and the maple syrup into the pudding, if desired.

Per serving: Calories: 291 Protein: 5g Carbs: 39g Sugar: 11g Fat: 14g

Feta Omelet With Roasted Tomato Sauce

SERVES 2 / PREP TIME: 5 MINUTES / COOK TIME: 1 HOUR INCLUDING SAUCE

This saucy take on the traditional omelet is sure to surprise your taste buds.

---

2 tbsp olive oil
3 beef tomatoes, sliced
1 sprig fresh thyme
1 sprig fresh rosemary
A pinch of salt and pepper to taste
1/2 tsp stevia powder

1 tbsp garlic-infused olive oil
10 egg whites
A pinch of salt to taste
1 tbsp chopped fresh parsley
1 tbsp garlic infused oil
2 oz crumbled feta cheese

---

1. Preheat the oven to 400 degrees.
2. Oil the bottom of a 9x13 baking dish with half of the olive oil.
3. Arrange the sliced tomatoes in this dish in a single layer.
4. Tuck the thyme and rosemary sprigs in among the tomato slices.
5. Sprinkle the tomatoes with the salt, the pepper, and the stevia.
6. Drizzle the rest of the olive oil and the garlic infused oil over the tomatoes.
7. Roast the tomatoes in the hot oven, uncovered, for 40-50 minutes.
8. When the tomatoes are done roasting, remove the thyme and rosemary sprigs.
9. Tip the entire contents of the dish into a food processor.
10. Blend until the tomatoes are smooth, then pour the sauce through a strainer into a clean frying pan.
11. Start the omelet by cracking the egg whites into a clean bowl.
12. Beat them with a whisk or fork before adding the salt and parsley.
13. Heat the garlic oil in a wide non-stick frying pan over medium heat.
14. Add the eggs to the pan and turn the heat to low for 10 minutes.
15. Next, lift the edges of the omelet slightly to make sure it easily lifts away from the pan.
16. Sprinkle the crumbled feta over the face of the omelet.
17. Take a spatula and lift one side of the omelet so that you can fold it over.
18. To serve, cut the omelet in half and place each side on a plate with a spoonful of the roasted tomato sauce.

Per serving: Calories: 453 Protein: 25g Carbs: 15g Fiber: 4g Sugar: 11g Fat: 34g

Herby Green Onion Scrambled Eggs

SERVES 4 / PREP TIME: 5 MINUTES / COOK TIME: 10 MINUTES

This herby variation on the breakfast classic makes the perfect brunch dish!

---

1 tsp coconut oil
4 egg whites
A pinch of salt to taste
1 tbsp fresh basil
1 tbsp sliced green onion (green tips)
To serve:
2 gluten free English muffins
2 large tomatoes, halved

---

1. Heat the oil in a skillet over medium-low heat.
2. Whisk together the salt, basil, green onion, and egg whites.
3. Once the oil is melted, pour the egg white mixture into the pan.
4. Cook for 10 minutes on low heat.
5. Stir continuously with a non-stick spatula.
6. Meanwhile, roast the tomato halves under a broiler set on low for about 5 minutes.
7. Cut the muffins in half and toast them in the toaster or in the broiler alongside the tomatoes.
8. Layer each plate with the scrambled eggs and tomato, placing a muffin half on the side.

Hint: If you want the eggs to cook faster, you can keep the heat on medium-low.

Tip: If you don't want to waste yolks, try buying a carton of pasteurized egg whites.

Per serving: Calories: 158 Protein: 7 Carbs: 27 Sugar: 5 Fat: 2

Smoked Salmon with Hash Brown Cakes

SERVES 4 / PREP TIME: OVERNIGHT / COOK TIME: 10 MINUTES

This delightful breakfast dish will satisfy your craving for locks and bagels.

---

1 1/2 medium white potatoes, peeled
1/4 tsp paprika
1 tbsp golden flax meal
1 tbsp coconut oil
Olive oil cooking spray
4 slices smoked salmon
2 tbsp capers

---

1. Boil the potatoes whole in 4 cups water until soft, about 20 minutes.
2. Drain well and set aside to cool.
3. When the potatoes are cool enough to handle, grate them on the coarse side of a cheese grater into a mixing bowl.
4. Add to the grated potatoes the paprika, the flax meal, and the coconut oil (you may need to use your hands to melt the coconut oil before mixing).
5. Mix well with a large spoon.
6. Divide the potato mixture into 4 equal balls by hand.
7. On a plate, pat each ball into a flat round.
8. Leave plate covered in the fridge overnight.
9. When you're ready to cook the cakes, heat a non-stick frying pan over medium heat and spray with olive oil cooking spray.
10. Gently fry the potato cakes 2 at a time.
11. Cook for 2 to 3 minutes on each side, or until they are light brown and heated through.
12. To serve, place 1 potato cake on each plate and top it with 1 slice of smoked salmon.
13. Sprinkle the capers over the salmon and serve.

Hint: Keep the potato cakes warm while you wait for the next batch to cook by placing them in a 200 degree oven.

Per serving: Calories: 215 Protein: 19g Carbs: 15g Fiber: 3g Sugar: 1g Fat: 9g

Homemade Gluten Free Everyday Bread

SERVES 8 / PREP TIME: 10 MINUTES / COOK TIME: 1 HOUR

Once you try this gluten free bread, it might just become your go-to bread recipe!

Coconut oil as needed
1 1/2 cups rice flour
1/2 cup buckwheat flour
3 tsp baking powder
1/2 tsp salt

2 tbsp coconut sugar
2 egg whites
1 cup unsweetened light coconut milk
1/2 cup coconut oil
2 tbsp sesame seeds

---

1. Preheat the oven to 350 degrees.
2. Grease a loaf pan generously with coconut oil.
3. Sift together the rice flour, the buckwheat flour, the baking powder, and the salt into a large bowl.
4. Stir in the sugar.
5. Meanwhile, using an electric mixer, lightly beat the egg whites until they are just frothy.
6. Stir in the milk and the coconut oil.
7. Now pour the flour mixture into the bowl with the egg white mixture.
8. Beat on a medium speed for 2 to 3 minutes, or until smooth.
9. Pour this mixture into the greased loaf pan.
10. Smooth the top with a spatula.
11. Next, sprinkle the sesame seeds over the top of the mixture, pressing them down slightly.
12. Bake for 55 minutes to 1 hour, testing to see if a toothpick or knife comes out clean.
13. Set the pan to cool on a wire rack for at least 10 minutes.
14. Turn the bread out onto the wire rack to finish cooling.

Hint: You can substitute other gluten free flours in place of the rice flour if you'd like.

Per serving: Calories: 268   Protein: 6g Carbs: 37g Sugar: 3g Fat: 18g

Fresh Buckwheat Blinis with Scrambled Eggs and Smoked Salmon

SERVES 4 / PREP TIME: 10 MINUTES / COOK TIME: 15 MINUTES

This hearty yet classy breakfast will satisfy the whole family!

3/8 cup buckwheat flour
1 tsp baking powder
A pinch of salt and pepper to taste
5/8 cup unsweetened rice milk
1 tbsp chopped green onions (green tips only)
2 egg whites

2 tsp coconut oil
4 large egg whites
To serve
2 tbsp capers
9 oz smoked salmon, sliced
4 wedges of fresh lime

---

1. For the blini batter, mix together the buckwheat flour, baking powder, salt and pepper, and rice milk to make a smooth batter.
2. Sprinkle in the green onions and mix until well combined.
3. In a separate bowl, whisk the first 2 egg whites with a pinch of salt until soft peaks form.
4. Gradually fold the whisked egg whites into the blini batter using a metal spoon.
5. Meanwhile, drizzle a small amount of the coconut oil into a frying pan over medium-high heat.
6. Spoon large tablespoons of the batter into the pan to make medium sized pancakes, about 4 inches in diameter.
7. Cook the blinis in batches for 2-3 minutes on the first side and 1-2 minutes on the other side, or until golden brown.
8. Repeat until all of the mixture is used up.
9. Keep the finished blinis warm by placing them on a tray in a 200-degree oven.
10. For the scrambled eggs, whisk the remaining egg whites in a bowl.
11. Drizzle the rest of the coconut oil into the frying pan.
12. Pour in the eggs and constantly stir with a spatula to cook and scramble the eggs.
13. To serve, place two blinis onto each of the four plates, spoon on the scrambled eggs, and sprinkle on a few capers.
14. Arrange the smoked salmon on the top and add the lime wedges.

Hint: Flip the blini pancakes when small bubbles appear on the surface. The underside should be a light golden color.

Per serving: Calories: 268 Protein: 24g Carbs: 20g Sugar: 1g Fat: 11g

Blueberry Breakfast Coffee Cake

SERVES 6 / PREP TIME: 3 HOURS TO CHILL / COOK TIME: 55 MINUTES

This delicious yet healthy breakfast cake is perfect for mid-morning brunch!

---

1 tbsp coconut oil
6 slices gluten free bread (try our Everyday Gluten Free Bread recipe)
1/2 cup organic blueberries (fresh or frozen)
8 large egg whites
1 1/8 cup unsweetened rice milk
1 tsp ground ginger

1 tsp vanilla extract
1/4 cup coconut sugar
1/4 cup coconut sugar
3 tbsp rice flour
1/2 tsp ground ginger
1 tbsp pure maple syrup

---

1. Grease a 9x13 baking dish with the coconut oil.
2. Cut the bread into 1 inch cubes.
3. Spread the cubes evenly over the bottom of the dish.
4. Sprinkle the blueberries over the bread.
5. Set aside.
6. Meanwhile, in a large bowl, whisk the egg whites, rice milk, ginger, vanilla extract, and 1/4 cup coconut sugar together until no lumps remain.
7. Pour this mixture evenly over the bread and blueberries.
8. Wrap the dish tightly with plastic wrap, or cover it with a lid, and refrigerate it for at least 3 hours, or overnight.
9. When you're ready to bake, preheat the oven to 350 degrees.
10. Remove the dish from the refrigerator.
11. Prepare the topping by whisking together 1/4 cup coconut sugar, rice flour, and ginger in a medium bowl until there are no lumps.
12. Sprinkle this topping evenly over the top of the bread.
13. Place the dish in the middle of the oven and bake for 45-55 minutes, or until golden brown on top.
14. For a crunchy topping, place the dish under the broiler on high for 2 to 3 minutes after it is done baking.
15. Drizzle a little maple syrup over each serving.
16. Cover any leftovers and refrigerate for up to 4 days.

Hint: You can add any topping you desire, such as low FODMAP fresh fruit.

Per serving: Calories: 248 Protein: 10g Carbs: 46g Sugar: 22g Fat: 5g

Chocolate Oat Gluten Free Waffles

SERVES 4 / PREP TIME: 20 MINUTES / COOK TIME: 15 MINUTES

These delicious waffles will satisfy your craving for a sweet treat anytime.

---

1 1/4 cup unsweetened light coconut milk
1 tbsp apple cider vinegar
1/4 cup melted coconut oil
2 tbsp pure maple syrup
1 tsp vanilla extract
1/4 cup steel cut oats (gluten free)
2 tbsp flax seeds
3/4 cup rice flour

1/2 cup potato starch
3 tsp baking cocoa powder
1/2 tsp salt
1 1/2 tsp baking powder
1/2 tsp ground ginger
2 tbsp coconut sugar

---

1. In a mixing bowl, combine the milk and the vinegar and let this sit for a few minutes so it can activate.
2. Whisk the rest of the wet ingredients into this mixture: the melted coconut oil, maple syrup, and vanilla extract.
3. In another bowl, whisk together the dry ingredients.
4. Pour the wet ingredients into the dry ingredients.
5. Stir it all together with a mixing spoon until just combined. The batter will still be a little lumpy.
6. Let the batter rest for 10 minutes so the flour has time to soak up some of the moisture.
7. Plug in your waffle iron to preheat now.
8. Once 10 minutes has passed, give the batter one more swirl with your spoon.
9. Pour some batter onto the heated waffle iron, enough to cover the center and most of the central surface area, and close the lid.
10. Once the waffle is crisp, transfer it to a cooling rack or baking sheet.
11. Don't stack your waffles on top of each other, or they'll lose crispness.
12. Repeat with remaining batter.

Hint: Keep your waffles warm by placing them on a rack in a 200 degree oven until you're ready to serve.

Per serving: Calories: 429 Protein: 5 Carbs: 59 Sugar: 13 Fat: 22

Nutty Cinnamon-Oat Granola Bars

SERVES 12 / PREP TIME: 10 MINUTES / COOK TIME: 40 MINUTES

These homemade granola bars are full of healthy fats to give you lots of energy.

1/2 cup coconut oil, melted
2 cups old fashioned rolled oats
1/2 cup sunflower seeds
1/4 cup sesame seeds
1/4 cup chopped pecans
3 tbsp pure maple syrup
1/2 cup coconut sugar
1 tsp ground ginger

---

1. Heat the oven to 325 degrees.
2. Grease a loaf baking pan with some of the coconut oil.
3. Mix together the oats, seeds, and nuts on a baking sheet.
4. Put the baking sheet in the oven for 5-10 minutes to toast.
5. Meanwhile, pour the rest of the coconut oil, the maple syrup, and the coconut sugar in a medium sized saucepan.
6. Heat the oil mixture over low heat, stirring until the oil is melted.
7. Turn the burner off.
8. Add the oat mix and ginger to the saucepan.
9. Now mix everything together until all the oats are well coated.
10. Pour this mixture into the loaf pan.
11. Press down lightly.
12. Bake for 30 minutes.
13. Once it's done, take the pan out of the oven and let it cool on a wire rack.
14. Once it's cool, cut the loaf into 12 bars.

Per serving: Calories: 562 Protein: 15g Carbs: 34g Sugar: 13g Fat: 44g

Mediterranean Grilled Cheese and Tuna

SERVES 2 / PREP TIME: 5 MINUTES / COOK TIME: 5 MINUTES

These open sandwiches are the perfect lunchtime treat.

---

1 (5 oz) can chunk light tuna in water
1 tbsp chopped chives (green tips only)
2 tbsp olive oil
A pinch of salt to taste
2 slices gluten free bread (try our Everyday Bread Recipe)

1 large tomato, sliced
1/2 cup goats cheese, crumbled
A pinch of paprika to serve

---

1. Turn on the broiler to high.
2. While the broiler is heating up, drain the tuna.
3. Flake the tuna into a medium bowl with a fork.
4. Add in the chives and olive oil.
5. Season with salt.
6. Meanwhile, toast the gluten free bread under the broiler until each slice is nicely browned on both sides, about 3 minutes total.
7. Remove the bread and spread the tuna mixture on top of each slice, right up to the edges of the toast.
8. Top each with a slice of tomato.
9. Sprinkle the cheese over the tomato.
10. Place the toast back under the broiler until the cheese is bubbling, about 1 minute.
11. Sprinkle each slice with a little paprika to serve.

Per serving: Calories: 342 Protein: 16 Carbs: 21 Sugar: 3 Fat: 22

Blueberry Orange Muffins

SERVES 12 / PREP TIME: 10 MINUTES /COOK TIME: 25 MINUTES

Delicious, fruity gluten free muffins.

1 1/4 cups gluten free all-purpose baking flour
2 tsp baking powder
3/4 cup unsalted coconut oil, softened
4 large egg whites
1 cup coconut sugar
3 tbsp almond milk

½ cup carob powder
Zest of 1 medium orange
1 1/2 cups organic blueberries

1. Heat oven to 350 degrees.
2. Line a 12-hole muffin tin with paper or foil muffin liners.
3. Pour all the ingredients except the fruit into a large bowl.
4. Beat the ingredients with an electric whisk on a medium speed until smooth.
5. Fold the fruit through the batter with a spatula by hand.
6. Fill each muffin paper about halfway.
7. Bake for 20-25 minutes, or until golden and just firm.
8. Remove the muffins from the oven and allow to cool on a wire rack.

Hint: Allow about 30 minutes for the muffins to cool enough to peel the papers in order to prevent the muffins from crumbling.

Per serving: Calories: 259 Protein: 3g Carbs: 37g Sugar: 23g Fat: 13g

Mediterranean Grilled Flat Bread

SERVES 1 / PREP TIME: 5 MINUTES / COOK TIME: 15 MINUTES

Be transported to the Middle East with this easy tomato and cheese lunchtime pita.

1 small zucchini, thinly sliced
2 tsp olive oil
1 dash dried basil
1 dash dried oregano
1 gluten free pita
1 roma tomato, sliced
1/4 cup mozzarella, grated

2 tbsp crumbled goats cheese
1 handful fresh basil leaves

1. Heat the oven to 425 degrees.
2. Meanwhile, place a frying pan over high heat on the stove top.
3. Toss the zucchini slices in a small bowl with the olive oil, the dried basil, and the oregano.
4. Lay the zucchini slices in the frying pan and cook for a few minutes on each side, or until tender.
5. Place the gluten free pita on a baking sheet.
6. Cover the pita with tomato slices.
7. Arrange the zucchini slices on top of the tomatoes.
8. Sprinkle the mozzarella and goats cheese over the tomatoes.
9. Place the pita in the oven and bake for 8 minutes, or until the cheese has melted and the pita's edges are crisp.
10. Garnish with a few basil leaves to serve.

Per serving: Calories: 404 Protein: 20g Carbs: 68g Sugar: 7g Fat: 24g

Quinoa Breakfast Falafel

SERVES 4 / PREP TIME: 10 MINUTES / COOK TIME: 30 MINUTES

This gluten-free version of the Middle Eastern classic is sure to delight your tastebuds.

1 cup quinoa
2 1/4 cups low FODMAP vegetable stock, hot
3 cups fresh spinach, leaves roughly chopped
½ cup gluten free breadcrumbs

1 1/2 cups feta cheese, cubed
2 large egg whites, beaten
2 tbsp olive oil
Romaine lettuce, to serve

1. Place the quinoa in a saucepan with the hot vegetable stock.
2. Simmer the quinoa for 18-20 minutes over a gentle heat, or until the grains have fluffed up and the liquid has disappeared.
3. Remove from the heat.
4. Stir in the spinach with the quinoa and allow the pan to cool.
5. Once it has cooled down, pour the quinoa and spinach into a medium bowl.
6. Add the breadcrumbs, the feta, and the egg whites, stirring thoroughly.
7. Set this mixture aside.
8. Meanwhile, gently heat the olive oil in a shallow frying pan.
9. Using your hands, form the quinoa mixture into 8 round patties.
10. Add these patties to the frying pan and fry for 4-5 minutes on each side, or until each one is crisp and golden.
11. Serve on a bed of romaine lettuce.

Hint: Stuff the falafel into a gluten free pita if you wish.

Per serving: Calories: 462 Protein: 20 Carbs: 41 Fiber: 5 Sugar: 5 Fat: 24 (Unsaturated: 12 Saturated: 11)

Mashed Potato Pancakes

SERVES 4 / PREP TIME: 10 MINUTES / COOK TIME: 30 MINUTES

Creamy mashed potatoes are transformed into crunchy cakes in this simple recipe.

Water to cover potatoes
2 small potatoes, peeled
4 tsp unsweetened rice milk
1 oz potato flakes
3 egg whites
1 tbsp goats milk

A pinch of salt to taste
1 dash paprika
Coconut oil for frying

1. Place the potatoes in a saucepan.
2. Fill the pan with water, enough to submerge the potatoes.
3. Bring the water to a boil over high heat.
4. Boil the potatoes until they are soft all the way through, about 20 minutes.
5. When they are done, drain the potatoes well and return them to the pan.
6. Add the rice milk.
7. Mash the potatoes well.
8. Stir in the potato flakes.
9. Gradually add the egg whites.
10. Now stir in the goats milk.
11. Next, season the potatoes with the salt, and paprika.
12. Warm a frying pan over medium heat and grease it with a little coconut oil.
13. When the oil is hot, pour a ladle of the potato mixture into the pan and cook for 5 minutes, or until golden around the edges.
14. Turn over the potato cake and cook for another 3 minutes, or until golden-brown.
15. Repeat with the remaining potato mixture.

Per serving: Calories: 139 Protein: 6g Carbs: 21 Sugar: 1g Fat: 4g

Gluten Free Savory Chicken Crêpes

SERVES 4 / PREP TIME: 10 MINUTES / COOK TIME: 40 MINUTES

This classic French dish comes to life with a delicious savory chicken filling.

---

2 tbsp olive oil
2 chicken breasts
3 tbsp buckwheat flour
1 1/2 unsweetened light coconut milk
1 handful fresh parsley, chopped
1 cup rice flour

1/2 tsp sea salt
4 large egg whites, plus one egg white beaten, for brushing
½ cup rice milk
1/3 cup gluten free breadcrumbs
1/2 cup lettuce, to serve

---

1. Heat 1 tbsp oil in a large frying pan and cook the chicken breasts for 5-8 minutes on each side, or until golden brown and cooked through. Set to one side.
2. In the same pan, stir in the buckwheat flour.
3. Now pour in the coconut milk, a little at a time, whisking continuously until you have a smooth sauce and allow to bubble for 2-3 minutes, or until thick.
4. Meanwhile, chop the chicken into pieces and add back to the pan along with any juices from the plate.
5. Stir in the parsley, turn off the heat and set aside.
6. To make the crêpes, pour the rice flour into a large bowl and whisk in the salt.
7. Make a well in the centre of the flour and pour in 2 egg whites.
8. Pour the rice milk over the flour and egg whites.
9. Now whisk the eggs and milk, working the flour into the liquid until you have a smooth, thin batter.
10. Heat a large non-stick frying pan or crêpe pan with a drizzle of oil.
11. When the pan is hot, pour in a ladle of the batter and quickly swirl the pan to spread it across the surface and cook for one or two minutes.
12. When the underside of the pancake is golden, flip it and cook it for 30 seconds.
13. Transfer the crêpe to a plate and make three more pancakes in the same way.
14. Heat oven to 400 degrees and line two cookie sheets with parchment paper.
15. Take one crêpe and brush a circle of beaten egg around the edge.
16. Pile a quarter of the chicken mixture into the centre of the crêpe.
17. Now fold the pancake over and press the edges together to make a calzone shape. Transfer crêpes to the cookie sheet as you complete each one.
18. Brush the top of each closed crêpe with egg.
19. Sprinkle the gluten free breadcrumbs over the crêpes and bake for 20-25 minutes, rotating the trays halfway through.
20. Serve on a plate with a side of lettuce.

Per serving: Calories: 407 Protein: 26g Carbs: 44g Sugar: 1g Fat: 15g

Italian Turkey Breakfast Patties

SERVES 4 / PREP TIME: 10 MINUTES / COOK TIME: 10 MINUTES

A perfect Sunday morning breakfast!

---

1 lb ground turkey
4 oz feta cheese
2 tbsp fresh basil
2 tbsp fresh oregano
½ lemon, zest only
2 egg whites
A pinch of salt to taste
2 tbsp rice flour
2 tbsp coconut oil
1/2 romaine lettuce to serve

---

1. For the patties, place all of the ingredients except the flour, oil and lettuce in a food processor.
2. Pulse these ingredients until well combined.
3. Using damp hands, shape the mixture into two patties.
4. Now dust the patties with the flour.
5. Heat the coconut oil in a frying pan over medium heat.
6. Fry the patties for 3-4 minutes on each side, or until golden-brown and cooked through.
7. Serve with a side of crispy romaine lettuce.

Per serving: Calories: 285 Protein: 31.5g Carbs: 6.5g Fiber: 1g Sugar: 1.5g Fat: 15g

Teatime Banana Bread

SERVES 8 / PREP TIME: 10 MINUTES / COOK TIME: 45 MINUTES

This naturally sweet bread is also perfect as an afternoon treat with tea.

---

1 large over-ripe banana
1 tbsp rice milk
1/4 cup coconut oil, softened
2/3 cup rice flour
1/3 cup coconut sugar
1/2 tsp baking soda
1/2 tsp baking powder

2 egg whites
1 dash vanilla extract

---

1. Preheat the oven to 325 degrees.
2. Grease or line a loaf baking pan with parchment paper.
3. Use a fork to mash the banana in a medium mixing bowl.
4. Add the remaining ingredients.
5. Beat the batter with an electric whisk until it is combined and smooth.
6. Spoon the mixture into the prepared loaf tin.
7. Level the top of the batter with a spoon or rubber spatula.
8. Bake for 40-45 minutes, or until the bread has risen, is shrinking away from the sides of the pan, and golden brown.
9. Set aside the bread to cool for 10 minutes.
10. Remove the banana bread from the pan and leave to cool on a wire rack.
11. Slice and serve.

Per serving: Calories: 137 Protein: 1g Carbs: 21g Sugar: 9g Fat: 6g

Carrot and Banana Breakfast Bars

SERVES 8 / PREP TIME: 10 MINUTES / COOK TIME: 45 MINUTES

This easy baked breakfast treat makes the perfect grab-and-go morning meal.

---

1 ripe banana, peeled, pitted, and mashed
3 tbsp pure maple syrup
1/4 cup coconut sugar
3 cups old fashioned rolled oats (gluten free)
2 medium carrots, grated
Zest of 1 orange
1/3 cup pumpkin seeds

---

1. Heat the oven to 325 degrees.
2. Line an 8x8 square baking dish with parchment paper.
3. Mix together the banana, the maple syrup, and the coconut sugar until it is smooth.
4. Mix in the rolled oats, the carrots, the orange zest, and the pumpkin seeds.
5. Stir everything well.
6. Next, pack the batter into the prepared pan, pushing down firmly.
7. Bake for 40-45 minutes.
8. Let the loaf cool in the pan before slicing into 8 bars.

Per serving: Calories: 203 Protein: 6g Carbs: 38g Sugar: 13g Fat: 4g

Traditional Lemon Poppy Seed Muffins

SERVES 6 / PREP TIME: 10 MINUTES / COOK TIME: 25 MINUTES

These gluten and lactose free classic muffins is simply tasty.

---

1 cup rice flour
1 tsp baking powder
1/2 tsp baking soda
A pinch of salt
Zest of 1 lemon
1/2 tbsp coconut oil, melted
1 egg white, room temperature
1/2 tsp vanilla extract
1/2 almond extract

1/4 cup pure maple syrup
1/4 cup cottage cheese
2 tbsp lemon juice
2 tbsp almond milk
2 tbsp poppy seeds

---

1. Heat the oven to 350 degrees.
2. Mix together the rice flour, baking powder, baking soda, salt and lemon zest in a mixing bowl.
3. In a separate bowl, whisk together the coconut oil, egg white, and vanilla extract.
4. Stir in the maple syrup and the cottage cheese until you get a smooth mixture.
5. Now stir in the lemon juice.
6. Stir the flour mixture into the liquid mixture until everything is just combined.
7. Pour in the milk while stirring.
8. Fold in the poppy seeds.
9. Divide the batter into six muffin cups.
10. Bake them 20-25 minutes in the oven.
11. Leave the muffins to cool in the pan for 10 minutes.
12. Remove from the pan and leave to cool for 5 minutes.

Hint: The muffins are done when a toothpick comes out clean. You can store the muffins for 5 days in the fridge.

Per serving: Calories: 174 Protein: 4g Carbs: 33g Fiber: 1g Sugar: 10g Fat: 3g

Savory Cilantro Oatmeal

SERVES 2 / PREP TIME: 5 MINUTES / COOK TIME: 10 MINUTES

A savory take on a classic breakfast - great if you don't have a sweet tooth!

---

1 cup unsweetened light coconut milk
1/4 cup steel cut oats (gluten-free)
A pinch of salt to taste
1/4 cup goat cheese, crumbled
1/2 tbsp fresh parsley
1 tsp fresh cilantro, loosely chopped

---

1. Pour the milk and the oats together into a small pan.
2. Bring the oats and milk to a boil.
3. Leave the oatmeal to simmer on low heat for 1-3 minutes, stirring now and then.
4. Leave the pan to warm up for a few minutes.
5. Season with salt.
6. Divide the savory oats into two bowls and crumble the goats cheese on top of each.
7. Finish with fresh parsley and cilantro.

Per serving: Calories: 163 Protein: 6g Carbs: 10g Sugar: 1g Fat: 12g

SEAFOOD

Shrimp Kebabs

SERVES 3 / PREP TIME: 10 MINUTES / COOK TIME: 10 MINUTES

Chunky grilled shrimp.

12oz shrimp, shelled
1 tsp dried oregano
1 tbsp garlic-infused olive oil, divided
3 tbsp fresh lemon juice
A pinch of salt and pepper
1 green bell pepper, roughly chopped

---

1. In a bowl stir together the shrimp, oregano, and half the olive oil, and marinate for as long as you've got (preferably at least one hour).
2. Whisk the remaining olive oil, lemon juice, salt and pepper in a separate bowl and place to one side.
3. Thread shrimp and green pepper pieces onto metal skewers and grill over medium-high heat in grill pan just for 2 minutes per side or until cooked through.
4. Serve with the olive oil and lemon dressing.

Per serving: Calories: 199 Protein: 29g Carbs: 4g Fiber: 1g Sugar: 1g Fat: 7g

Clam Chowder

SERVES 6 / PREP TIME: 20 MINUTES / COOK TIME: 1 HOUR

A traditional home made dish.

---

1 tbsp olive oil
2 large carrots, peeled and diced
1/2 cup rice flour
2 cups low FODMAP seafood stock
2 cups rice milk
12 oz clams, shucked and chopped
1/2 tsp white pepper

1 tbsp dried parsley
1 bay leaf
12 small potatoes, peeled and diced into 1 inch cubes

A pinch of salt and pepper

---

1. In a large stockpot heat the oil over medium heat. Add the carrots and sauté for 5 minutes.
2. Gradually sift in the flour, stirring thoroughly and scraping the bottom of the pan.
3. Next slowly stir in the seafood stock, making sure there are no lumps.
4. Stir in rice milk until mixture is smooth.
5. Add the clams and spices, bring soup to a boil, then cover and reduce heat.
6. Simmer for 30 minutes.
7. Add diced potatoes, cover and simmer for an additional 30 minutes.
8. Season with salt and pepper to taste.

Per serving: Calories: 221 Protein: 11g Carbs: 36g Fiber: 3g Sugar: 5g Fat: 4g

Thai Rice Noodle Salad

SERVES 3 / PREP TIME: 5 MINUTES / COOK TIME: 10 MINUTES

Fresh ingredients and a crisp taste.

Dressing: 2 tbsp fish sauce 1 tbsp white vinegar 2 tbsp fresh lime juice	1 tbsp garlic infused oil 8oz shrimp, shelled and de-veined 1 cup flat, 1/4 inch dry rice noodles 1/4 cup peeled, diced, seeded cucumber 1/4 cup scallions, sliced 1 tbsp fresh cilantro leaves, finely chopped 1 tbsp fresh mint leaves, finely chopped 1/4 cup pineapple, diced (canned or fresh)

1. Prepare your dressing by combining all ingredients in a small bowl and place to one side.
2. Add the oil to a skillet on medium heat.
3. Sauté the shrimp for 5-6 minutes or until thoroughly cooked through.
4. Cook the rice noodles according to package directions.
5. Now mix the rest of the ingredients in a salad bowl.
6. Drain the noodles and stir through the salad ingredients.
7. Top with the shrimp and drizzle with the dressing.
8. Serve!

Per serving: Calories: 409 Protein: 17g Carbs: 69g Fiber: 4g Sugar: 3g Fat: 6g

Classic Calamari and Tilapia Paella

SERVES 4 / PREP TIME: 10 MINUTES / COOK TIME: 1 HOUR

This scrumptious blend of seafood is sure to please anyone craving paella!

---

3 tbsp garlic-infused olive oil
7 oz calamari (squid), cut into round strips
2 cups water
1 cup dry white wine
1 cup brown rice
1 (6 oz) tilapia fillet, cut into big squares
A pinch of salt
2 tbsp turmeric
½ cup freshly chopped parsley (plus more to sprinkle on top)
4 oz cooked chicken breast, cut into small pieces

---

1. Heat the olive oil in a large, deep pan over medium-high heat.
2. To the warm pan, add the calamari and cook for 5-10 minutes, or until the squid turns white or pink.
3. Stir the calamari frequently while cooking.
4. Next, add in the water and the wine and bring it to a boil.
5. Let this cook for 30 minutes over medium heat.
6. Now add the rice, tilapia, salt, turmeric, parsley, and chicken breast.
7. Bring all of this to a boil, then reduce the heat to low.
8. Simmer this pot for 30 minutes, or until the water is almost absorbed and the rice is tender.
9. Remove from the heat and serve with freshly chopped parsley sprinkled on top.

Per serving: Calories: 426 Protein: 28g Carbs: 36g Fiber: 3g Sugar: 1g Fat: 14g

Tuna, Carrot and Zucchini Fritters

SERVES 3 / PREP TIME: 10 MINUTES / COOK TIME: 10 MINUTES

These lightly fried bites are tasty and satisfying.

1/2 medium zucchini, grated
½ (5 oz) can tuna
1 medium potato, peeled, boiled and cubed
1/2 medium carrot, peeled and grated
¼ cup chives (green tops only), chopped

1 tbsp capers
A pinch of salt to taste
1/4 tsp lemon pepper
1 tbsp brown rice flour
1 egg white
3 tbsp coconut oil

---

1. Grate the zucchini in a colander over the sink.
2. Press on the zucchini in the colander to drain the water.
3. In a large bowl, combine the tuna, potatoes, grated carrot, zucchini, chives, capers, salt, and lemon pepper, and gently mix.
4. Add the flour and egg, combining it all together.
5. Heat the coconut oil in a large skillet over medium-high heat.
6. Scoop a big tablespoon of batter into the oil for each fritter.
7. Flatten the batter with a spatula.
8. Cook and flip until all sides are nice and golden brown, about 2 minutes for each side.
9. Serve immediately.

Per serving: Calories: 235 Protein: 12g Carbs: 16g Fiber: 2g Sugar: 2g Fat: 14g

Savory Fish and Potato Winter Stew

SERVES 3 / PREP TIME: 10 MINUTES / COOK TIME: 50 MINUTES

This delicious stew is the perfect way to stay warm on a cold evening.

---

4 tbsp coconut oil
1 bay leaf
3 medium potatoes, peeled and sliced into half-inch thick slices
1 red bell pepper, seeded and sliced
2 large tomatoes, diced
1 lb cod fillet, cut into strips
1 cup water

1 cup dry white wine
3 tbsp fresh oregano, chopped
A pinch of sea salt
A pinch of dried parsley
1 tsp turmeric
1/2 tsp paprika

---

1. Heat the coconut oil and the bay leaf in a large deep pan over medium-high heat.
2. Reduce the heat to medium.
3. Add a layer of potatoes, a second layer of bell peppers, and a third layer of tomatoes.
4. Lay the cod strips on top.
5. Add the water and the wine so you can bring it to a boil.
6. As it is reaching boiling point, sprinkle the stew with the oregano, sea salt, parsley, turmeric, and paprika.
7. Simmer the stew for 40 minutes, or until potatoes are done.
8. Remove from the heat and serve in deep bowls.

Per serving: Calories: 523 Protein: 27g Carbs: 47g Fiber: 7g Sugar: 7g Fat: 19g

Quinoa Tuna Sandwich Spread

SERVES 4 / PREP TIME: 10 MINUTES / COOK TIME: 20 MINUTES

If you like quinoa and tuna, this hearty tuna spread is perfect for lunch any day.

2 cups water
1 cup quinoa
A pinch of sea salt
1 cup fresh or frozen spinach
¼ cup chives (green tips only)
3 (5 oz) cans light tuna in water
1 tbsp lemon juice
1 tbsp lime juice

A pinch of sea salt
1 tbsp olive oil

1. Bring the water to a boil in a saucepan over high heat.
2. Add the quinoa and a pinch of salt to the boiling water.
3. Cook the quinoa for 15 minutes.
4. Now add the spinach and reduce the heat to low.
5. When the water is gone, turn off the heat.
6. Fluff the quinoa and spinach with a fork.
7. Meanwhile, mix the chives with the tuna.
8. Now combine the quinoa and spinach with the tuna.
9. Add the lemon juice, lime juice, salt, and olive oil.
10. To serve, spread over a gluten free cracker or a piece of gluten free toast.

Per serving (spread only): Calories: 258 Protein: 22g Carbs: 28g Fiber: 4g Sugar: 1g Fat: 7g

Lime and Parsley Encrusted Cod

SERVES 2 / PREP TIME: 10 MINUTES / COOK TIME: 25 MINUTES

This zesty breadcrumbed cod makes the perfect light summer dish.

---

2 (6 oz) cod fillets
1/2 slice gluten free bread, toasted and crumbled into breadcrumbs
3 tbsp fresh parsley, finely chopped
1 tbsp garlic-infused olive oil
Zest of 1/2 lime
1 squeeze of lime juice
A pinch of salt and pepper to taste
Lime wedges to serve

---

1. Heat the oven to 425 degrees.
2. Lay out your cod fillets in a shallow, oven-proof dish.
3. In a bowl, mix the breadcrumbs together with the parsley, garlic infused oil, lime zest, lime juice, salt, and pepper.
4. Mix thoroughly with your fingers.
5. Pour the seasoned breadcrumbs over the cod and press the crumbs firmly onto the cod to form an even crust on both sides.
6. Bake for 20-25 minutes, or until the crust is browned and the fish is flaky and white.
7. Serve immediately, with lime wedges on the side.

Per serving: Calories: 191 Protein: 25g Carbs: 4g Fiber: 1g Sugar: 0g Fat: 8g

Lemon and Oat Crusted Salmon

SERVES 2 / PREP TIME: 10 MINUTES / COOK TIME: 10 MINUTES

Delicious with a side of greens.

---

2 large egg whites
1 1/2 cups quick-cooking oats (gluten-free)
1 tsp paprika
2 (6 oz) fresh salmon fillets
2 tbsp coconut oil
A pinch of salt to taste
2 lemon wedges

---

1. Whisk the egg whites in a shallow dish.
2. Combine the oats and the paprika in a separate shallow dish.
3. Now dip the salmon fillets into the egg whites, coating both sides.
4. Then dip the salmon into the oat mixture.
5. Press the oats gently into both sides of the salmon to form a sturdy crust.
6. Place the coated fillets on greased baking sheet.
7. Once you have finished coating the salmon, discard the oat mixture to prevent contamination.
8. Heat the coconut oil in a large, non-stick skillet over medium-high heat.
9. Add the fillets to the oil once it is hot.
10. Cook the salmon for 4 to 5 minutes on each side, or until it flakes easily when tested with a fork.
11. Season the salmon with a pinch of salt to taste.
12. Serve each fillet with a wedge of lemon.

Hint: To further prevent sticking, lay a sheet of parchment paper down instead of greasing the baking sheet.

Per serving: Calories: 595 Protein: 45g Carbs: 42g Fiber: 7g Sugar: 1g Fat: 27g

Spicy Oriental Cod Cakes

SERVES 2 / PREP TIME: 10 MINUTES / COOK TIME: 15 MINUTES

Deliciously fragrant fish cakes.

---

1 (12 oz) cod fillet, cooked and shredded
1 egg white
1 tsp minced lemongrass
½ tsp minced ginger
1 tsp oyster sauce
1 tsp chopped fresh cilantro

2 tsp fresh parsley, loosely chopped
Coconut oil for frying
Lime wedges to serve

---

1. Place the cod in the bowl of a food processor or blender with the egg white.
2. Process until the cod and egg white are roughly combined (don't over do this, use the pulse setting if you have one for around 10-20 seconds).
3. Transfer this mixture to a large bowl.
4. To the bowl, add the minced lemongrass, ginger, oyster sauce, cilantro, and parsley. (You can add these ingredients to the processor in order to mince if you wish.)
5. Mix everything together until well combined.
6. Using damp hands, roll the mixture into balls the size of a tablespoon.
7. Flatten each ball slightly.
8. Add enough coconut oil to a wok to reach a depth of 2 inches.
9. Heat the wok over medium-high heat until a tiny piece of bread sizzles when you drop it in.
10. Add 5 or 6 cod cakes to the hot oil.
11. Cook each cake for 3 minutes, or until golden.
12. Use a slotted spoon to transfer the cakes to a plate lined with a paper towel.
13. Repeat in batches with the remaining fish cakes.
14. Serve the cakes with lime wedges.

Hint: You can also check that the oil is hot enough by dropping in one grain of rice. It will rise to the top and start cooking.

Per serving: Calories: 594 Protein: 26g Carbs: 2g Fiber: 0g Sugar: 1g Fat: 55g

Baked Lime Sea Bass

SERVES 4 / PREP TIME: 10 MINUTES / COOK TIME: 25 MINUTES

This easy yet tasty recipe will spice up any large white fish.

---

1 (3 lb) sea bass, gutted and cleaned
3 lemongrass stalks, cut diagonally into
2½ cm pieces
1 (1 inch) piece fresh ginger, peeled and
sliced
2 tbsp garlic-infused olive oil

2 limes

---

1. Preheat the oven to 400 degrees.
2. Wash the sea bass inside and out, and pat it dry with a paper towel.
3. Score lines across the fillet and through the skin 4-5 times on each side.
4. Now lay the fish on a large piece of oiled aluminum foil (big enough to wrap up the fillet loosely).
5. Put the lemongrass, and ginger into a mortar with 1 tablespoon of the garlic oil.
6. Squeeze the juice of one of the limes into the mortar bowl.
7. Mash the ingredients in the mortar with a pestle just until everything is bruised.
8. Next, pour out half the pounded mixture over the fish.
9. Add the last of the garlic oil to the fish as well.
10. Rub everything in, making sure you push some mixture into the cuts.
11. Cut the second lime into quarters.
12. Push two pieces of the lime into the bass's cavity along with the remainder of the pounded mixture.
13. Squeeze the juice from the last two lime quarters over the fish.
14. Pull the sides of the foil up to create a loose packet.
15. Crimp the edges of the foil to seal it, making sure there is some space around the fish.
16. Bake for 25 minutes.
17. After baking, let it rest for about 5 minutes before opening the packet.
18. Try serving with your choice of rice or low FODMAP vegetables.

Per serving: Calories: 416 Protein: 64g Carbs: 6g Sugar: 2g Fat: 14g

Lime Cod En Papillote

SERVES 4 / PREP TIME: 10 MINUTES / COOK TIME: 12 MINUTES

Individual foil packets create the perfect steaming environment in this take on "en papillote."

---

2 stalks lemongrass, peeled and bruised
¼ cup chives (green tips only), sliced
2 tbsp chopped fresh cilantro
4 (6 oz) cod fillets
1 lime, juiced
1 tbsp fish sauce
A pinch of salt and pepper to taste
2 tbsp olive oil

---

1. Preheat the oven to 425 degrees.
2. Place a large, oven-proof frying pan in the oven to preheat.
3. Place four large squares of aluminum foil on the work surface.
4. Place an equal amount of lemongrass, chives and cilantro on each piece of paper.
5. Place the fillets on top of each square.
6. Pour the lime juice and fish sauce over everything.
7. Season each fillet with salt and pepper to taste.
8. Finally, place half a tablespoon of oil on top of each fillet.
9. Fold the foil over to encase the ingredients, crimping the edges down to create a seal.
10. Make sure that there is room for steam to circulate in the foil packets.
11. Remove the heated frying pan from the oven.
12. Place the foil packets in the pan.
13. Put the pan in the oven for 12 minutes.
14. After baking, allow the packets to cool for about 5 minutes before opening them.

Hint: Instead of the frying pan, you could preheat a roasting pan in the oven.

Per serving: Calories: 183 Protein: 25g Carbs: 4g Fiber: 0g Sugar: 2g Fat: 7g

Classic Steamed Bass with Lime and Brown Rice

SERVES 4 / PREP TIME: 10 MINUTES / COOK TIME: 20 MINUTES

The rice wine, ginger and garlic adds a taste of the Orient to this sea bass recipe.

---

1 cup Swiss chard
4 (5 oz) sea bass fillets
1 tbsp ginger, finely shredded
1 tbsp garlic-infused olive oil
1 tsp rice wine
1 bunch green onions, finely shredded
(green tips only)
2 tbsp fresh cilantro, chopped
2 cups brown rice, cooked to serve
1 lime, cut into wedges, to serve

---

1. Preheat the oven to 400 degrees.
2. Tear off a large rectangle of foil, big enough to make a large envelope.
3. On the foil, place the Swiss chard, the sea bass, the ginger, and the garlic oil.
4. Pour the rice wine over this.
5. Fold the foil over and seal the edges by crimping them.
6. Put it on a baking sheet.
7. Bake for 20 minutes.
8. After it's done baking, open the parcel and scatter the green onions and cilantro over the fish.
9. Serve with brown rice and lime wedges on the side.

Per serving: Calories: 284 Protein: 31g Carbs: 25g Sugar: 1 Fat: 6g

Greek Tilapia Bream with Yellow Squash

SERVES 2 / PREP TIME: 30 MINUTES / COOK TIME: 20 MINUTES

This marinated delight is perfect any night of the week.

---

2 (6 oz) tilapia fillets
1 lemon, juiced
2 tbsp olive oil, plus extra for drizzling
1 tbsp capers
1 can (2oz) anchovies
2 large tomatoes, halved
A pinch of salt to taste

1 tbsp fresh parsley, finely chopped
A pinch of dried oregano
1 tbsp fresh mint, finely chopped
2 small yellow squash
2 cups fresh spinach leaves

---

1. For the bream, place the tilapia fillets in a bowl.
2. Squeeze the lemon juice over the fish.
3. Leave to marinate for 30 minutes.
4. Meanwhile, preheat the oven to 400 degrees.
5. Heat 1 tbsp olive oil in a large frying pan over medium heat.
6. Add the capers and anchovies.
7. Cook for 5 minutes, or until the anchovies have dissolved.
8. Add in the tomatoes, squashing them slightly.
9. Season this with salt.
10. Cook for five minutes.
11. Now place the tilapia in an oven-proof dish.
12. Add in the parsley, the tomatoes, the juices from the pan, a drizzle of olive oil, and the oregano.
13. Cover it all with aluminum foil.
14. Bake this in the oven for 20 minutes, removing the foil halfway through cooking.
15. While the fish is baking, make the salad.
16. Whisk 1 tbsp olive oil with the mint in a small bowl and set aside.
17. Next, trim the ends of the squash.
18. With a potato peeler or mandolin, slice the squash lengthways into wafer-thin slices.
19. Add the squash slices to the dressing.
20. Mix it well.
21. Set the dressing aside to marinate for at least 10 minutes.
22. After it has marinated, mix the spinach with the squash.
23. Place the salad on dinner plates.
24. When the fish is cooked, let it rest for one minute.
25. Serve the fish alongside the salad.

Per serving: Calories: 308 Protein: 26g
Carbs: 14g Fiber: 4g Sugar: 8g Fat: 18g

Fresh Tuna and Salmon Ceviche

SERVES 4 / PREP TIME: 10 MINUTES / COOK TIME: NA CHILL TIME: 30 MINUTES

The fresh take on ceviche is sure to delight everyone.

1 (6 oz) skinless salmon fillet, flesh sliced as thinly as possible
1 (6 oz) skinless tuna fillet, flesh sliced as thinly as possible
5 limes, juice and zest
4 tbsp olive oil
1 handful fresh cilantro leaves, loosely chopped

1 large seaweed paper, crushed and shredded, to serve
Olive oil to serve
4 lime wedges to serve

1. Put the fish slices into a large, shallow serving bowl.
2. Mix gently, using your fingers.
3. Sprinkle the lime zest over the fish.
4. In a separate bowl, whisk together the lime juice and olive oil until well combined to make a marinade.
5. Pour the marinade over the fish.
6. Again, mix gently using your hands.
7. Cover the bowl with plastic wrap.
8. Chill the bowl in the fridge for at least 30 minutes.
9. When ready to serve, mix in the chopped cilantro.
10. To serve, place one egg ring into the center of each of four serving plates.
11. Spoon in enough ceviche to almost reach the top of the egg rings.
12. Top with the shreds of seaweed paper and a drizzle of olive oil.
13. Garnish the plate with a wedge of lime.
14. Carefully remove the egg rings before serving.

Per serving: Calories: 305 Protein: 22g Carbs: 14g Fiber: 1g Sugar: 3g Fat: 19g

Monk fish Medallions with Lemon Dressing

SERVES 4 / PREP TIME: 20 MINUTES / COOK TIME: 15 MINUTES

Marinated meaty fish makes this dish one to return to again and again.

---

4 (5 oz) boneless monkfish medallions
1 stalk lemongrass, bruised and finely chopped
4 fresh lime leaves, chopped
1 tsp fresh lemon thyme leaves, chopped
5 tbsp olive oil, plus extra for frying
A pinch of salt to taste
2 lemons, zest only
2 tbsp coconut sugar

1/2 cup water
3 tbsp olive oil
2 tsp lemon juice
½ tsp coriander seeds, toasted and ground
½ tsp chopped green onions, green tips only
2 tbsp roughly chopped fresh cilantro
1 handful spinach to serve

---

1. Place the monkfish in a bowl with the lemongrass, lime leaves, lemon thyme leaves, olive oil, and salt.
2. Cover and chill for as long as possible.
3. Meanwhile, make the lemon dressing.
4. Chop the strips of lemon zest into a small dice.
5. Throw the zest into a pan of boiling water.
6. Drain the boiling water off the zest once it has returned to a rolling boil.
7. In a small saucepan, pour in the blanched lemon zest, coconut sugar, and water.
8. Cook this sugar mixture for about 5 minutes.
9. Now drain the lemon zest.
10. In a medium bowl, mix the sweetened zest together with the lemon juice, coriander seeds, green onion, cilantro, and 2 tablespoons of water.
11. About 20 minutes before you're ready to eat, remove the monkfish from the marinade.
12. Lightly season it with salt and pepper.
13. Heat a drizzle of olive oil in a large non-stick frying pan over medium heat.
14. Fry the monkfish medallions for 4 minutes on each side, or until golden brown.
15. Remove the cooked medallions from the pan and allow them to rest in a warm place for 4 minutes.
16. Serve with the dressing and spinach.

Hint: Serve the monkfish on top of cooked brown rice to add to the meal.

Per serving: Calories: 376   Protein: 25g Carbs: 8g Sugar: 6g Fat: 29g

Moroccan Tilapia and Tomato Tagine

SERVES 6 / PREP TIME: 10 MINUTES / COOK TIME: 20 MINUTES

The delicious sweetness of Moroccan cooking is featured in this fun tilapia recipe.

---

1 tbsp olive oil
2 tsp grated fresh ginger
1 tsp ground cumin
1 tsp turmeric
1 cinnamon stick
1 (15 oz) can diced tomatoes
1 dash salt
1 cup water
1 lb (of 2 oz) tilapia fillets
2 tsp pure maple syrup

1 tbsp chopped green onions (green tips only)
1 squeeze lemon juice to serve

---

1. Heat the olive oil in a large frying pan over medium heat.
2. Add the ginger, cumin, turmeric, and cinnamon stick.
3. Cook the spices for two minutes, stirring regularly.
4. Now add the tomatoes, salt, and the water.
5. Cook, stirring frequently, for 10 minutes.
6. Add the tilapia and simmer for 5 minutes, or until the fish is almost cooked through and tender.
7. Add the maple syrup and green onions and cook 2-3 more minutes.
8. To serve, spoon out the tagine into bowls.
9. Give each bowl a squeeze of lemon juice to serve.

Hint: Traditional tagine is cooked in a tagine clay dish. You can pick these up from homeware shops and add to the authenticity and taste of the meal if you can get hold of one!

Per serving: Calories: 117 Protein: 15g Carbs: 5g Fiber: 2g Sugar: 3g Fat: 5g

Oriental Shrimp Pasta

SERVES 4 / PREP TIME: 10 MINUTES / COOK TIME: 20 MINUTES

Fresh and fast to cook and so scrumptious!

---

5 tbsp reduced sodium soy sauce
3 tbsp coconut sugar
3 tbsp fresh lime juice
2 tbsp rice vinegar
2 tsp sesame oil
2 cups carrots, sliced thinly
1 tbsp chopped fresh ginger
6 green onions, green tips only, sliced
Olive oil cooking spray

5 oz fresh spinach leaves
1 1/4 lb medium raw shrimp, peeled and de-veined
1/4 tsp salt
12 fl oz water (or double the amount of noodles)
8 oz rice noodles

---

1. In a medium bowl, whisk together the first four ingredients.
2. Set this mixture aside.
3. Heat the sesame oil in a large skillet on medium-high heat.
4. Add the carrots and continue cooking until they are tender, about 4 minutes.
5. Add the ginger and about three-quarters of the green onions and cook for 1 minute, stirring frequently.
6. Transfer the ginger and onions to a medium bowl.
7. Return the skillet to the stove top and mist it with cooking spray over medium heat.
8. Add the spinach and cook until wilted, stirring frequently, 2 to 3 minutes.
9. Add this to the bowl with the carrot mixture.
10. Return the skillet to the stove top and mist it with cooking spray over medium heat again.
11. Toss in the shrimp and a pinch of salt to taste.
12. Cook, turning occasionally, until the shrimp are firm to the touch and opaque in the thickest part, or about 4 to 6 minutes.
13. Meanwhile, bring a large pot of water to a boil.
14. Add the rice noodles and cook, stirring frequently, until al dente, about 3 minutes, then drain the water.
15. Give the soy sauce mixture a quick whisk.
16. Add the soy sauce to the noodles.
17. Heat the noodles and sauce to a simmer over medium-high heat.
18. Reduce the heat to medium and add the carrot mixture.
19. Gently toss everything together until it is all combined and heated through. Stir in the shrimp.
20. Serve right away, garnishing with the remaining green onions.

Per serving: Calories: 394 Protein: 24g
Carbs: 63g Fiber: 5g Sugar: 7g Fat: 4g

Lime Shrimp Fritters

SERVES 4 / PREP TIME: 20 MINUTES / COOK TIME: 20 MINUTES

These zesty fritters are complemented perfectly with this homemade lime dressing.

---

1 lb large raw shrimp, peeled, de-veined
and rinsed
2 egg whites, beaten
2 tbsp chives, green tips only, diced
2 tbsp lime juice
2 cups gluten free bread crumbs
1 lime, juice and zest
1/8 tsp sea salt
2 tbsp olive oil

---

1. In a food processor, pulse the shrimp to coarsely chop it.
2. Add the egg whites, chives and lime juice.
3. Pulse everything together to combine.
4. Add 1 cup the bread crumbs, pulsing to combine.
5. Remove the mixture and form into balls with your palms.
6. Roll the balls in the remaining 1 cup bread crumbs to coat.
7. Place the balls on a parchment-lined baking sheet.
8. Refrigerate for 10 minutes.
9. While the shrimp balls rest, whisk together 1 tbsp the olive oil, lime juice, lime zest, and sea salt.
10. In a large non-stick pan, heat the rest of the olive oil over medium-high heat.
11. Working in batches, fry the fritters until they are golden brown, or about 4 minutes per side.
12. Serve the fritters hot with the lime dressing.

Per serving: Calories: 584 Protein: 20g Carbs: 13g Fiber: 1g Sugar: 2g Fat: 50g

Grilled Sardines with Cilantro Brown Rice

SERVES 2 / PREP TIME: 30 MINUTES / COOK TIME: 20 MINUTES

A simple dish from pantry items, yet so tasty!

1 tbsp low sodium soy sauce
1 lime, juice
1 thumb-sized piece fresh ginger, grated
1 tsp garlic-infused olive oil

1 tbsp pure maple syrup
10 oz fresh sardines
1 cup brown rice
¼ cup scallions, sliced, green tips only
1 tbsp fresh cilantro, chopped

1. To make the marinade, mix together the soy sauce, lime juice, ginger, garlic oil, and maple syrup.
2. Pour the marinade over the sardines.
3. Cover the marinade and chill for 30 minutes.
4. Preheat the broiler on high when ready to cook.
5. Place the sardines, skin-side up, on a baking sheet lined with parchment paper.
6. Broil the sardines for 5 minutes.
7. Turn and baste them with the remaining marinade.
8. Broil for 5 more minutes.
9. Meanwhile, cook the rice following the package instructions.
10. After it's cooked and drained, toss the rice with the scallions and cilantro.
11. Serve the spicy rice with the sardines.

Per serving: Calories: 381 Protein: 23g Carbs: 45g Fiber: 3g Sugar: 9g Fat: 12g

Danish Potato Salad with Herring

SERVES 4 / PREP TIME: 10 MINUTES / COOK TIME: 20 MINUTES

Traditional herring salad with dill and lemon dressing.

1/2 cup water
2 lemons, juice only
1/2 cup white wine
2 bay leaves
1 tbsp white wine vinegar
1 tsp salt
4 oz herring fillet
4 cooked small potatoes

4 tbsp olive oil
1 tbsp chopped fresh dill
1/2 lemon, juice only
A pinch of salt to taste
3 sprigs fresh dill to serve
Lemon wedges to serve

---

1. First, bring the water, lemon juice, white wine, bay leaves, white wine vinegar, and salt to a slow boil in a pan.
2. Turn down the heat to a gentle simmer.
3. Add the herring to the pan.
4. Poach it for about 12 minutes, or until cooked through.
5. For the potato salad, cut the cooked potatoes in half.
6. Place them into a large bowl.
7. In another bowl, combine the olive oil, dill, lemon juice, and salt.
8. Add this mixture to the bowl with the potatoes.
9. Stir to coat the potatoes.
10. Meanwhile, drain the fish and flake.
11. Stir into the potato salad, garnish with more dill and the lemon wedges to serve.

Per serving: Calories: 333 Protein: 7g Carbs: 19g Fiber: 2g Sugar: 2g Fat: 23g

Grilled Tomato Salad with Mackerel and Capers

SERVES 4 / PREP TIME: 5 MINUTES / COOK TIME: 15 MINUTES

This fast and simple salad is the perfect lunch.

---

4 large tomatoes, halved
1 tbsp capers, drained
1/2 cup feta cheese, crumbled
1 cup fresh spinach leaves, washed
15 oz canned mackerel, drained and
sauce reserved
1 tbsp olive oil
1 tbsp red wine vinegar
A pinch of salt to taste

---

1. Preheat the broiler on high.
2. Place the halved tomatoes (skin side up) on a baking tray covered in parchment paper.
3. Broil for 5-10 minutes, or until lightly chargrilled.
4. After removing the tomatoes from the oven, sprinkle over the capers and feta.
5. Meanwhile, divide the spinach among 4 plates.
6. Roughly break up the mackerel and add it to the spinach already on the plates.
7. Place the tomato halves on top of the mackerel.
8. Then mix together the oil and vinegar in a small bowl.
9. Drizzle this over the tomatoes.
10. Sprinkle with a pinch of salt to taste and serve.

Per serving: Calories: 261 Protein: 25g Carbs: 7g Fiber: 2g Sugar: 4 Fat: 15g

Ginger Tempura Shrimp

SERVES 2 / PREP TIME: 30 MINUTES / COOK TIME: 5 MINUTES

This classic dish has been transformed into a gluten free treat.

---

1 tsp finely chopped fresh ginger
1 tbsp coconut sugar
½ tbsp rice vinegar
1 cup water
1/2 cup rice flour
A pinch of salt
1 cup club soda
10 large shrimp (peeled and butterflied)
Coconut oil for deep frying

---

1. For the dip, heat the ginger, coconut sugar, rice vinegar, and water in a saucepan over medium heat for 10-15 minutes.
2. Remove the dip from the heat and set aside until you are ready to use it.
3. To make the tempura, mix the rice flour and salt in a large bowl.
4. Gradually whisk in the club soda to form a smooth batter.
5. Set this aside for 20-30 minutes.
6. Next heat the coconut oil in a deep-fat fryer to 350 degrees.
7. Dip the shrimp into the batter.
8. Deep fry each shrimp in the hot oil for 1-2 minutes, or until golden brown and cooked through.
9. Serve the fried shrimp alongside the ginger dip.

Hint: CAUTION: Hot oil can be dangerous. Do not leave the fryer unattended.

Per serving: Calories: 465 Protein: 8g Carbs: 45g Fiber: 2g Sugar: 2 Fat: 29g

Ginger and Parsley Salmon Patties

SERVES 4/ PREP TIME: 10 MINUTES / COOK TIME: 10 MINUTES

A wonderful combination of herbs and spices.

---

4 (5 oz) boneless, skinless salmon fillets
1 thumb-sized piece fresh ginger, grated
1 lemon, juice
¼ cup fresh parsley, chopped
A pinch of salt to taste

1 tsp coconut oil
2 cups spinach leaves, washed
1 tbsp olive oil
1 cup cooked brown rice

---

1. Place the salmon in a food processor bowl with the ginger, half the lemon juice, the chopped parsley, and the salt.
2. Pulse until this mixture is roughly minced.
3. Shape the mixture into 4 patties.
4. Meanwhile, heat the oil in a non-stick frying pan over medium-high heat.
5. Fry the patties for 4-5 minutes on each side, turning until crisp and cooked through.
6. Combine the spinach leaves with the olive oil and the rest of the lemon juice.
7. Serve the patties with the cooked rice and spinach salad.

Per serving: Calories: 305 Protein: 32g Carbs: 13g Fiber: 1g Sugar: 1g Fat: 13g

Gluten-Free Tomato Pasta with Tuna

SERVES 4 / PREP TIME: 5 MINUTES / COOK TIME: 25 MINUTES

A family favorite!

---

3 tbsp olive oil
3 tbsp fresh parsley, chopped
1 thumb-sized piece fresh ginger, grated
3 medium tomatoes, diced
1 (6.5 oz) can tuna in oil, drained and flaked

1 tbsp garlic-infused olive oil
A pinch of salt to taste
1 ½ cups rice spaghetti noodles

---

1. To prepare the sauce, heat the oil in a saucepan.
2. Toss in 2 tablespoons of the parsley and the ginger.
3. Sauté for a few minutes.
4. Add in the tomatoes and cook for another few minutes.
5. Fold in the tuna, garlic oil, and a pinch of salt to taste.
6. Leave the sauce to simmer for 10 minutes.
7. Meanwhile, cook the rice spaghetti noodles for 8-10 minutes, or according to package directions.
8. Drain the pasta and return it to the pan.
9. Pour the tuna sauce into the pasta and toss well.
10. To serve, sprinkle the remaining parsley over the pasta.
11. Divide it among four bowls.

Per serving: Calories: 528 Protein: 15g Carbs: 75g Fiber: 4g Sugar: 2g Fat: 18g

Pan Grilled Tuna Steaks with Fresh Basil and Quinoa

SERVES 4 / PREP TIME: 8 MINUTES / COOK TIME: 20 MINUTES

This refreshing combination of tuna, basil, and quinoa is sure to be a winner.

---

2 cups water
1 cup quinoa
4 tbsp olive oil
1 tbsp red wine vinegar
2 tbsp finely chopped fresh basil
1 tsp smoked paprika
4 (5 oz) tuna steaks
4 tbsp olive oil
1 lemon, zest and juice
1 tbsp fresh parsley, chopped
A pinch of salt to taste

---

1. Bring the water to a boil in a pan over high heat.
2. Add the quinoa and lower the heat.
3. Cover and simmer the quinoa for 20 minutes, or until most of the water has been soaked up.
4. Meanwhile, whisk 1 tbsp olive oil, vinegar, basil, and smoked paprika together in a small bowl.
5. Now place the tuna steaks in a separate medium bowl with the other 3 tablespoons of olive oil, the lemon zest, the lemon juice, the parsley, and the salt (pour the juices into the pan for added flavor).
6. Heat a pan over medium-high heat.
7. Add the tuna steaks and fry on each side for 2-3 minutes, or until cooked through.
8. Turn off the heat to the quinoa and allow to steam with the lid on.
9. To serve, drizzle the dressing over the grilled tuna and serve on a bed of quinoa.

Per serving: Calories: 276 Protein: 20g Carbs: 14g Fiber: 2g Sugar: 1g Fat: 15g

Baked Herb Salmon with Lime

SERVES 8 / PREP TIME: 10 MINUTES / COOK TIME: 60 MINUTES

This delightful take on baked salmon allows you to cook a big meal without a lot of fuss.

---

4 1/2 lb salmon with skin on
3 limes, sliced
1/4 cup fresh parsley, chopped
2 tbsp fresh tarragon, chopped
2 bay leaves
2 tbsp chopped green onions (green tips only)
1 tbsp white wine

---

1. Preheat the oven to 400 degrees.
2. Place the salmon fillet, skin-side down, on a large sheet of foil or parchment paper.
3. Cover the salmon with the lime slices, herbs, and onions.
4. Splash the salmon with the wine.
5. Fold up the foil or paper and crimp the edges to seal up the packet.
6. Place on a baking sheet.
7. Bake the salmon for 50 minutes to 1 hour, or until cooked through.
8. Check the salmon by poking a knife into the fillets and making sure the flesh flakes easily.
9. Slice the fish into portions and serve with your choice of low FODMAP vegetables or rice.

Per serving: Calories: 379 Protein: 55g Carbs: 3g Fiber: 1g Sugar: 1g Fat: 15g

Mint and Dill Baked Salmon

SERVES 4 /   PREP TIME: 10 MINUTES /   COOK TIME: 20 MINUTES

The olive and dill salsa verde on this salmon is delicious!

1/4 cup fresh dill, roughly chopped
1/4 cup fresh mint, roughly chopped
1/4 cup fresh parsley, roughly chopped
1/4 cup green onion(green tips only),
roughly chopped
2 tbsp capers
2 lemons, juice only
4 small salmon fillets, skin on
1 cup white basmati rice

---

1. Preheat the oven to 400 degrees.
2. To make the salsa verde, put the herbs, onions, capers, and the juice of 1 ½ of the lemons into a food processor.
3. Pulse until the mixture is roughly chopped.
4. Meanwhile, place the salmon fillets onto a lightly oiled baking sheet.
5. Squeeze the juice of the remaining lemon half over the fish.
6. Bake the fish in the oven for 10-12 minutes, or until cooked through.
7. While the fish is baking, cook the rice according to the package instructions.
8. To serve, pile the salsa verde on top of the salmon fillets with the rice on the side.

Per serving: Calories: 282 Protein: 27g Carbs: 15g Fiber: 2g Sugar: 1 g Fat: 13g

Fish Tacos

SERVES 4 / PREP TIME: 5 MINUTES / COOK TIME: 15 MINUTES

A lighter alternative to the usual beef tacos.

10oz skinless cod fillet, halved
½ tsp ground cumin
A pinch of salt and pepper to taste
1 tbsp garlic-infused olive oil
1 tbsp olive oil
1 lime juice and zest
4 rice tortillas
½ cup lettuce/spinach leaves, washed
¼ cup large beef tomatoes, diced

---

1. Season your fish with the cumin and the salt and pepper.
2. Set the fish to one side.
3. Heat the oil in a skillet over medium heat.
4. Add the cod.
5. Cook each side for 5 minutes.
6. Meanwhile, use a small dish to mix together the olive oil, lime zest and juice.
7. You can heat up your tortillas in the microwave or under the broiler on low.
8. Once the fish is cooked, flake with a fork.
9. Layer the tortillas with lettuce, tomato, and fish.
10. Drizzle your lime dressing over your fish tortillas, roll and enjoy!

Per serving: Calories: 349 Protein: 26g Carbs: 27g Fiber: 4g Sugar: 3g Fat: 16g

Maple and Dill Salmon

SERVES 2 / PREP TIME: 5 MINUTES / COOK TIME: 20 MINUTES

A wonderfully sweet and savory baked fish recipe.

A pinch of salt and pepper
1 tbsp maple syrup
2 5oz salmon fillets, skinless
1 lemon, halved
1 tbsp dried dill

---

1. Preheat oven to 400 degrees when ready to cook.
1. Combine the maple syrup, salt and pepper in a small bowl.
2. Marinade the salmon for as long as you can in this mixture.
3. Line an oven tray with foil or parchment paper.
4. Place the salmon fillets onto the foil.
5. Squeeze half the lemon juice over the salmon and fold the foil/paper into a parcel with the lemon wedges inside.
6. Bake in the oven for 15 to 20 minutes until thoroughly cooked through.
7. Remove from the oven and sprinkle over the dill.
8. Serve with your choice of salad, rice or vegetables.

Per serving: Calories: 246 Protein: 36g Carbs: 11g Fiber: 1g Sugar: 8 Fat: 6g

Coconut and Pineapple Shrimp

SERVES 2 / PREP TIME: 15 MINUTES / COOK TIME: 10 MINUTES

A delicious sweet and savory meal!

---

1 slice gluten free bread
½ cup unsweetened desiccated coconut
2 egg whites
12oz shrimp, peeled and de-veined (defrosted if frozen)

Pineapple Sauce:
¼ cup canned pineapple, diced
1 tbsp garlic-infused olive oil

---

1. Preheat oven to 400 degrees.
2. Line an oven tray with greaseproof parchment paper.
3. Make breadcrumbs out of the bread either with your fingers or in a blender.
4. Then, mix together the breads crumbs with the coconut in a shallow dish.
5. In a small bowl whisk the egg whites.
6. Dip each shrimp into the egg whites followed by the coconut breadcrumbs.
7. Transfer each shrimp to the oven tray and bake in the oven for 5 minutes on each side.
8. Meanwhile, heat the garlic oil in a skillet over medium heat.
9. Add the pineapple chunks and sauté for 5 minutes or until hot through.
10. Allow to cool slightly.
11. Serve immediately once cooked through with the pineapple sauce.

Per serving: Calories: 535 Protein: 49g Carbs: 33g Fiber: 5g Sugar: 19 Fat: 23g

Lime Crab Cakes

SERVES 4 / PREP TIME: 10 MINUTES / COOK TIME: 20 MINUTES

So refreshing!

---

3 slices gluten free bread
16oz cooked crab meat
½ tsp dried basil
½ tsp dried oregano
½ tsp marjoram
½ tsp dried parsley
A pinch of salt and pepper
2 egg whites

---

1. Preheat oven to 400 degrees.
2. Line an oven tray with greaseproof parchment paper.
3. Make breadcrumbs out of the bread either with your fingers or in a blender.
4. Mix with the rest of the ingredients in a mixing bowl.
5. Slightly wet your hands and use your palms to shape 2 fish cakes.
6. Bake in the oven for 10 minutes on each side.
7. Serve with your choice of salad.

Per serving: Calories: 135 Protein: 24g Carbs: 10g Fiber: 1g Sugar: 1g Fat: 2g

Crayfish and Lemon

SERVES 2 / PREP TIME: 10 MINUTES / COOK TIME: 10 MINUTES

Deliciously simple!

---

2 lemons, juiced
1 tbsp garlic-infused olive oil
1 tbsp fresh parsley
A pinch of salt and pepper
2 crayfish/lobster tails

---

1. Preheat the broiler to medium heat.
2. Whisk together the lemon, oil, parsley and salt and pepper (keep lemon wedges).
3. Place tails on a baking sheet.
4. With a sharp knife or kitchen shears, carefully cut top side of shells lengthways.
5. Pull apart shells slightly, and season meat with the oil dressing.
6. Broil the tails 5 to 10 minutes or until meat is opaque.
7. Garnish with lemon wedges to serve.

Per serving: Calories: 121 Protein: 12g Carbs: 3g Fiber: 1g Sugar: 1g Fat: 7g

POULTRY

Turkey Vegetable Rice Soup

SERVES 4 / PREP TIME: 5 MINUTES / COOK TIME: 8 HOURS IN SLOW COOKER

A restoring recipe!

---

2 medium carrots, peeled and copped
1 medium zucchini, chopped
1/2 cup celery stalks, sliced
2 large potatoes, chopped
4 (5oz) boneless and skinless turkey breasts
1 tsp olive oil
4 cups low FODMAP chicken stock

1 cup water
¾ cup brown rice
½ tsp dried thyme
A pinch of salt and pepper to taste
1 tbsp fresh cilantro/parsley
1 lemon, juice

---

1. Add all of the ingredients (Except for the lemon juice and herbs) into the slow cooker.
2. Cook on low for 7-8 hours or until the turkey is thoroughly cooked through.
3. Stir in the lemon juice and then turn off the slow cooker.
4. Ladle into individual bowls to serve and top with a sprinkle of fresh cilantro/parsley.

Per serving: Calories: 224 Protein: 9g Carbs: 45g Fiber: 5g Sugar:4 Fat: 2g

Chicken Burgers and Pineapple

SERVES 2 / PREP TIME: 5 MINUTES / COOK TIME: 20 MINUTES

A delicious combination of lean meat burgers with zesty pineapple!

---

1 tbsp canola oil

For the burgers:
10oz lean ground chicken breast (or turkey)
1 tbsp dried dill
1 lemon, juice
½ tsp dried thyme
A pinch of salt and pepper

For the salad:

½ cup canned pineapple, diced
¼ cucumber, diced
¼ cup salad lettuce (check individual tolerance with lettuce)
1 tbsp olive oil
A pinch of salt and pepper

---

1. In a large mixing bowl, combine all of the ingredients for the burgers and mix well.
2. Use slightly wet palms to form 2 burger patties.
3. Heat the canola oil in a skillet over medium-high heat.
4. Add the burgers, cooking for 3-4 minutes before turning and allowing to cook on the other side for a further 8-10 minutes or until thoroughly cooked through (check with a knife in the center of each burger to ensure there is no pink meat and that juices run clear).
5. Now combine all of the salad ingredients in a salad bowl and toss to coat.
6. Serve each burger with a helping of side salad and enjoy!

Hint: make up extra burgers and freeze in separate zip lock bags for 2-3 weeks – simply defrost before cooking thoroughly.

Per serving: Calories: 416 Protein: 43g Carbs: 10g Fiber: 2g Sugar: 6g Fat: 23g

Thai Spiced Chicken Noodle Stock

SERVES 4 / PREP TIME: 5 MINUTES / COOK TIME: 20 MINUTES

Our favorite pick-me-up with a little extra bounce!

2 cups water
2 cups low FODMAP chicken stock
8oz/1 cup gluten free noodles
2 (5 oz) cooked chicken breasts, skinless and boneless
½ cup celery, sliced
2 medium carrots, sliced
1 lime leaf

1 tsp dried basil
1 tsp dried cilantro
A pinch of salt and pepper to taste
1 cup bok choy
1 lime, juice and zest

1. Add the water and chicken stock into a large pot over high heat and bring to the boil, stirring frequently.
2. Lower the heat slightly and add the gluten free noodles, chicken and vegetables into the pot.
3. Bring to a simmer and then reduce the heat down to low.
4. Add the herbs and salt and pepper to taste.
5. After 10 minutes add the bok choy leaves and lime juice.
6. Cook for 5 minutes or until leaves are slightly wilted.
7. Stir through the lime zest and ladle into soup bowls to serve.

Per serving: Calories: 244 Protein: 5g Carbs: 53g Fiber: 3g Sugar: 2g Fat: 1g

Loaded Potato Skins

SERVES 2 / PREP TIME: 5 MINUTES / COOK TIME: 50 MINUTES

These are a perfect dinner time meal for the whole family!

---

2 large white potatoes, sliced in half
1 tbsp garlic-infused olive oil
A pinch of salt and pepper
4oz cooked chicken breast, skinless
and boneless
2 tbsp chives, chopped
1 red pepper, finely diced
2 tbsp goats cheese, crumbled

---

1. Preheat oven to 350 degrees.
2. Place the potatoes in a deep casserole dish.
3. Drizzle the garlic-infused olive oil on top of each half and season with salt and pepper.
4. Bake in the oven for 30-40 minutes or until skins are crispy and potato is fluffy and soft.
5. Remove from the oven and allow to cool.
6. Scoop out the potato from the inside and add to a mixing bowl.
7. Leave the skins to one side.
8. Add the chopped cooked chicken, chives, and diced pepper to the potato and mix well.
9. Scoop this mixture back into the potato skins and place back in the oven.
10. Cook for a further 10 minutes or until golden and sprinkle with goats cheese until bubbling and crispy.
11. Remove and serve with a side salad of your choice.

Per serving: Calories: 391 Protein: 26g Carbs: 34g Fiber: 4g Sugar: 4g Fat: 17g

Lemon and Cilantro Chicken Salad

SERVES 2 / PREP TIME: 10 MINUTES / COOK TIME: 15 MINUTES

A light summer dish or delicious side.

---

2 (5 oz) skinless and boneless chicken breasts
1 lemon, juiced
1 tbsp olive oil
1 tsp dried oregano
1 tsp dried thyme
A pinch of salt and pepper

For the salad:
2 large tomatoes, sliced
½ cucumber, sliced
2 scallions stems, sliced (green tips only)

1 tbsp fresh cilantro, chopped
2 cups spinach, washed (organic if possible)
1 tbsp olive oil
A pinch of salt and pepper

---

1. Preheat the broiler to medium-high heat.
2. Butterfly each chicken breast and flatten.
3. Mix 1 tbsp olive oil, juice of ½ lemon, dried herbs and a little salt and pepper together to form your marinade.
4. Marinate the chicken for as long as possible (preferable overnight).
5. Add to a lined baking tray and broil for 10-12 minutes on each side.
6. Ensure chicken is cooked thoroughly by inserting a knife into the center – the juices should run clear and meat should be white.
7. Now combine the salad ingredients and toss to coat.
8. Slice the chicken breast and layer on top of the salad.

Per serving: Calories: 395 Protein: 45g Carbs: 11g Fiber: 4g Sugar: 5g Fat: 19g

Teriyaki Meatballs

SERVES 2 / PREP TIME: 10 MINUTES / COOK TIME: 35 MINUTES

A little Asian twist on an Italian favorite!

For the meatballs:
10oz lean ground turkey
1 egg white
1 tbsp gluten free bread crumbs (optional)
1 tsp dried rosemary
1 tbsp fresh ginger
2 scallion stems, sliced (green tips only)
1 tbsp reduced sodium soy sauce

For the sauce:
¼ cup reduced sodium soy sauce
½ cup water
1 red bell pepper, diced
2 tsp brown sugar
1 tbsp potato starch

1. Preheat oven to 350 degrees.
2. Lightly oil a baking tray.
3. In a medium bowl mix together the ingredients for the meatballs.
4. Then, form 10 meatballs with the palms of your hands.
5. Place the meatballs on the tray.
6. Bake the meatballs for 20 minutes or until they are fully cooked through (no pink meat left).
7. Stir together all of the ingredients for the sauce (excluding the starch) in a pan over medium heat.
8. Bring to a simmer and add your cooked meatballs to the sauce.
9. Cover and simmer in the sauce for 5 minutes.
10. Meanwhile stir 2 tbsp water into the potato starch in a separate small bowl.
11. Add this into the meatball sauce to thicken (you could add 1 tbsp rice flour at this stage instead to thicken).
12. Once the sauce is thick, serve right away over rice or noodles.

Per serving: Calories: 454 Protein: 43g Carbs: 19g Fiber: 2g Sugar: 8g Fat: 23g

Garlic Sautéed Chicken and Sunflower Sauce

SERVES 2 / PREP TIME: 5 MINUTES / COOK TIME: 1 HOUR

This easy one-pot meal is sure to please any guests with nut allergies.

---

3 tbsp garlic-infused olive oil
4 (5 oz) chicken breasts, skinless
Water to cover chicken
2/3 cup rice milk
2 tbsp sunflower butter
A pinch of salt

---

1. Heat the oil in a large pot over medium-high heat.
2. Toss in the chicken and cook for 4-5 minutes, or until golden brown, turning often to ensure even color.
3. Cover the chicken with water (just enough to submerge chicken) and leave to cook over medium-low heat for about 40 minutes, stirring occasionally.
4. In a separate bowl, whisk the milk and sunflower butter until well blended.
5. Add this mixture to the chicken, stir and leave for a further 20 minutes.
6. Give everything a good stir.
7. Salt this mixture to taste.
8. Remove from the heat and serve.

Hint: You may consider serving this with your favorite rice.

Per serving: Calories: 323 Protein: 33g Carbs: 4g Fiber: 1g Sugar: 3g Fat: 19g

Minty Chicken Noodle Soup

SERVES 6 / PREP TIME: 10 MINUTES / COOK TIME: 40 MINUTES

This take on the classic cold day soup is refreshing and tasty!

½ cup fresh or frozen spinach, chopped
2 carrots, peeled and sliced
6 cups low FODMAP chicken stock
6 (5 oz) skinless cooked chicken
breasts
1 cup rice vermicelli noodles
A pinch of salt
1 tbsp fresh mint leaves, chopped

---

1. In a large pot, add the spinach, carrots, and the stock.
2. Bring this to a simmer over medium-high heat.
3. Turn down the heat slightly and allow to simmer for 30 minutes.
4. Meanwhile, shred the chicken with forks or meat claws.
5. To the stock, add the noodles, shredded chicken, and salt.
6. Cook for 7 minutes.
7. Ladle in to bowls and serve with the mint leaves.

Per serving: Calories: 371 Protein: 33g Carbs: 42g Fiber: 2g Sugar: 0g Fat: 6g

Indian Chicken and Rice

SERVES 3 / PREP TIME: 10 MINUTES / COOK TIME: 1 HOUR

This simple yet scrumptious chicken and rice dish will have you asking for more!

---

3 tbsp garlic-infused olive oil
2 (5 oz) chicken breasts, skinless
1 tbsp turmeric
Water to cover chicken
1 cup white rice
1 large carrot, finely chopped
A pinch of sea salt

---

1. Heat the oil in a large non-stick frying pan over medium-high heat.
2. Toss in the chicken and turmeric and cook for 5-6 minutes, or until golden brown, turning often to ensure even color.
3. Cover the chicken with water (to just submerge chicken) and let it cook over medium heat for 20 minutes, stirring occasionally.
4. Add the rice and carrots.
5. Top up the water to cover the ingredients.
6. Bring to a boil over high heat.
7. Salt the soup to taste, then reduce the heat to low.
8. Cover and simmer for another 15 minutes, or until all the water is absorbed and the rice is tender.
9. Give everything a good final stir before removing from the heat.
10. Let the dish stand, covered, for 15 minutes before serving.

Per serving: Calories: 477 Protein: 26g Carbs: 54g Fiber: 2g Sugar: 0g Fat: 1g

Gluten Free Turkey and Tomato

SERVES 4 / PREP TIME: 5 MINUTES / COOK TIME: 15 MINUTES

Delight your guests with this tasty pasta dish.

---

2 (6 oz) turkey breasts
2 tbsp lemon juice
A pinch of salt
4 oz rice noodles
2 large tomatoes, quartered
¼ cup green onions (green tips only) sliced
1 squeeze lime juice

¼ cup sesame seeds
A pinch of salt to taste
1 tbsp olive oil to serve

---

1. Season the turkey with the lemon juice and a pinch of salt.
2. Sauté the turkey over medium heat for 3-5 minutes on each side, or until no longer pink.
3. Cut the turkey breasts in half.
4. Cook the noodles for 4 minutes in a bowl of boiling water.
5. Drain the noodles under cold water.
6. Transfer them to a salad bowl.
7. Stir in the tomatoes, green onions, and lime juice.
8. Sprinkle the sesame seeds over the noodles.
9. Finally, season the noodles to taste with the salt and olive oil.
10. Serve the turkey on a bed of noodles.

Per serving: Calories: 204 Protein: 11g Carbs: 28g Fiber: 3g Sugar: 2g Fat: 5g

Fresh Ginger Chicken Salad

SERVES 3 / PREP TIME: 10 MINUTES / COOK TIME: 30 MINUTES

This well-garnished and tasty salad will make you re-think salads for good!

---

1 1/2 tbsp coconut sugar
2/3 cup fresh lemon juice
1 inch piece fresh ginger, grated
5 lime leaves
1 lemongrass stalk, chopped
2 (5 oz) chicken breasts, cut into strips
1 carrot, peeled and grated
1 bunch bok choy, finely sliced
4 oz rice noodles, cooked

2 tbsp fresh cilantro leaves, chopped

---

1. For the dressing, place the sugar, lemon juice, and ginger in a saucepan and bring to a boil over high heat, stirring until the sugar has dissolved.
2. Add the lime leaves, and lemongrass.
3. Return the mixture to a boil.
4. Remove the pan from the heat and leave to cool.
5. When cool, strain the mixture through a fine mesh strainer and set aside.
6. Meanwhile, add the chicken to a parchment lined baking tray.
7. Place it under the broiler on medium heat for 15-20 minutes, or until completely cooked through.
8. Turn the chicken occasionally while it is broiling.
9. Meanwhile, mix the carrot, bok choy, and noodles together in a bowl.
10. Add the dressing and mix it all together until well combined.
11. Divide the salad between 2 serving bowls.
12. To serve, top the salad with the chicken pieces and sprinkle the cilantro on top.

Per serving: Calories: 434 Protein: 26g Carbs: 77g Fiber: 5g Sugar: 38g Fat: 3g

Roasted Herby Chicken and Potatoes

SERVES 6 / PREP TIME: 10 MINUTES / COOK TIME: 1 HOUR
This potato and chicken dish is sure to be a dinner winner!

3 cups red potatoes, thinly sliced
2 tbsp olive oil
6 (5oz) chicken breasts, skin on
1 lemon, sliced into wedges
5 sprigs fresh thyme (or 2 tbsp dried)

1 cup white wine
1 cup low FODMAP chicken stock

1. Preheat the oven to 425 degrees.
2. Place the potatoes into a 9x13 glass baking dish.
3. Drizzle them with 1 tbsp the oil.
4. Season to taste with salt and pepper.
5. Toss to coat the potatoes.
6. Roast the potatoes in the oven for 20 minutes, or until they start to crisp.
7. Add the chicken to the baking dish along with the lemon wedges and thyme.
8. Drizzle the chicken with the remaining oil.
9. Return the dish to the oven for 20 minutes.
10. Next, pour the wine and stock over the dish.
11. Roast for a final 20 minutes, or until the chicken is golden and cooked through.

Per serving: Calories: 476 Protein: 57g Carbs: 9g Fiber: 1g Sugar: 0g Fat: 19g

Herby Shrimp and Chicken Risotto

SERVES 4 / PREP TIME: 5 MINUTES / COOK TIME: 50 MINUTES

A hearty and wholesome low FODMAP risotto dish.

---

2 medium tomatoes, diced
1 tbsp olive oil
1 tbsp garlic-infused olive oil
3/4 cup risotto rice
4 (5 oz) skinless chicken breasts, halved
2 tsp chopped fresh rosemary
2 tsp chopped chives

4 cups low FODMAP chicken stock
A pinch of salt to taste
8 large raw shrimp

---

1. Preheat the oven to 425 degrees.
2. Place the diced tomatoes in the bottom of a baking dish.
3. Drizzle the garlic oil over the tomatoes.
4. Roast for 20 minutes, or until the tomatoes are softened.
5. Stir in the risotto rice, chicken, rosemary, chives, chicken stock, and salt, mixing well.
6. Return the dish to the oven for 20 minutes.
7. Remove the dish and stir in the shrimp.
8. Return to the oven for 10 more minutes, or until the rice is tender and the chicken and shrimp are thoroughly cooked through.

Per serving: Calories: 322 Protein: 39g Carbs: 14g Fiber: 1g Sugar: 2 Fat: 12g

Lime Chicken Kebabs

SERVES 2 / PREP TIME: 30 MINUTES / COOK TIME: 55 MINUTES

This healthy take on the Mediterranean favorite is sure to please everyone!

---

2 tbsp olive oil
1 tsp crushed coriander seeds
1 tsp grated lime zest
½ tsp coconut sugar
1 tbsp garlic-infused olive oil
2 (5 oz) chicken breasts, cubed
1 lime, cut into wedges
2 metal skewers

---

1. Preheat the oven to 375 degrees.
2. Mix together the ingredients for the marinade: the olive oil, the coriander seeds, the lime zest, the coconut sugar, and the garlic oil.
3. Set the marinade aside.
4. Place the cubed chicken breasts in a glass baking dish.
5. Spoon the marinade over the chicken.
6. Next, squeeze a little lime juice over the top.
7. Cover and marinate for 30 minutes in the fridge.
8. When ready to cook, thread the marinated chicken onto the skewers.
9. Place each loaded skewer onto a baking sheet.
10. Roast the chicken skewers, uncovered, for 20-25 minutes.
11. Serve the kebab with a side of freshly washed spinach or your choice of salad.

Per serving: Calories: 352 Protein: 31g Carbs: 2g Fiber: 1g Sugar: 1g Fat: 24g

Easy Orange Maple Chicken

SERVES 4 / PREP TIME: 10 MINUTES / COOK TIME: 20 MINUTES

A fresh and healthy citrus chicken dish.

---

4 (5 oz) skinless chicken breasts
3 tbsp pure maple syrup
1 orange, zest only
2 tbsp fresh orange juice
A pinch of salt to taste

---

1. Score each chicken breast with a sharp knife.
2. Place the rest of the ingredients into a wide, shallow bowl.
3. Mix well.
4. Add the chicken breasts to this mixture and stir to coat.
5. Marinade for as long as possible in the fridge.
6. When ready to cook, preheat the broiler to low.
7. Shake off any excess marinade from the chicken and place on a lined baking tray.
8. Broil the chicken breasts for 10 minutes on each side.
9. Turn them once and baste on the marinade half way through.
10. Bake until the chicken is brown and glossy.
11. Slice each chicken breast in half and serve with your choice of vegetable or rice.

Per serving: Calories: 206 Protein: 31g Carbs: 11g Fiber: 0g Sugar: 11g Fat: 4g

Roasted Red Pepper Chicken

SERVES 4 / PREP TIME: 10 MINUTES / COOK TIME: 40 MINUTES

This smoky baked chicken dish is sure to be a crowd pleaser!

---

2 (5 oz) skinless chicken breasts
2 red bell peppers, de-seeded and sliced
1 tbsp garlic-infused olive oil
1 tsp smoked paprika
3 tbsp olive oil
1 lemon, zest and juice
2 tbsp fresh basil, chopped
2 tbsp fresh cilantro, chopped

---

1. Preheat the oven to 400 degrees.
2. Place the chicken and peppers in a large bowl.
3. In another bowl, mix together the garlic infused oil, paprika, olive oil, lemon zest, and lemon juice.
4. Pour the marinade over the chicken and peppers and transfer to a lined baking sheet.
5. Roast the chicken for 40 minutes, turning over halfway through.
6. Bake until the chicken is cooked through and the juices run clear.
7. Serve the chicken and peppers in bowls with freshly torn basil and cilantro.

Per serving: Calories: 223 Protein: 16g Carbs: 4g Fiber: 1g Sugar: 3g Fat: 15g

Classic Chicken Meatballs and Rice

SERVES 2 / PREP TIME: 10 MINUTES / COOK TIME: 20 MINUTES

Our take on a Swedish favorite.

½ celery stalk, sliced
1 small carrot, peeled and sliced
2 (5 oz) skinless chicken breasts, sliced
2 tbsp chives (green tips only)
Coconut oil for greasing
1 cup cooked brown rice
A pinch of salt to taste

---

1. Preheat the oven to 400 degrees.
2. Blend the celery, carrot, chicken, and chives in a food processor until it is finely chopped together.
3. Shape into small meatballs with your palms.
4. To cook, put on a baking sheet lined with foil and greased with a little coconut oil.
5. Bake the meatballs for 20 minutes or until cooked through.
6. (Turn over halfway through baking).
7. Serve with the brown rice seasoned with the salt.

Hint: If cooking the brown rice at the same time as meatballs, add 2 cups water to a sauce pan with the rice over high heat and bring to the boil. Lower the heat to a simmer and cook for 20 minutes. Turn down the heat, drain any excess water, cover and steam for 5 minutes.

Per serving: Calories: 344 Protein: 34g Carbs: 25g Fiber: 3g Sugar: 2g Fat: 1g

Chicken Salad and Patatas Bravas

SERVES 4 / PREP TIME: 10 MINUTES / COOK TIME: 40 MINUTES

A clean and fresh salad with a Spanish twist.

---

2 baking potatoes, peeled and cubed
2 tbsp olive oil
2 tbsp smoked paprika
4 tsp balsamic vinegar
A pinch of salt to taste
1 red bell pepper, seeded and diced

4 (5 oz) skinless boneless chicken breasts
2 cups fresh spinach

---

1. Preheat the oven to 400 degrees.
2. Spread the potatoes onto a large baking sheet.
3. Mix 1 tbsp the oil with 1 tbsp the paprika, half the balsamic vinegar, and the salt.
4. Pour this mixture over the potatoes.
5. Toss the potatoes in the oil mixture until coated.
6. Bake in the oven for 10 minutes.
7. Meanwhile, prepare the chicken.
8. Mix the pepper with the chicken in a small bowl.
9. Sprinkle the chicken with the rest of the paprika.
10. Spread the chicken and peppers on top of the potatoes.
11. Return the dish to the oven for 30 minutes, or until the chicken is cooked and the potatoes are crispy.
12. When the chicken is cooked, mix together the remaining oil and balsamic vinegar.
13. Drizzle this over the spinach.
14. Serve the chicken with the paprika potatoes and spinach salad.

Per serving: Calories: 393 Protein: 36g Carbs: 37g Fiber: 6g Sugar: 4g Fat: 11g

Chicken and Tomato Stew

SERVES 4   PREP TIME: 10 MINUTES   COOK TIME: 45 MINUTES

A savory blend of tomatoes and parsley simmers with chicken breast in this hearty dish.

1 tbsp olive oil
4 (5 oz) skinless chicken breasts
1 stalk celery, finely chopped
1 medium carrot, peeled and finely diced
A pinch of salt
1 (15 oz) can diced tomatoes
1 cup low FODMAP chicken stock
1 tbsp tomato paste
1 tsp dried oregano

1 tbsp garlic-infused olive oil
1 tbsp chopped parsley to serve
1 tsp coconut sugar
2 cups potatoes, cubed

1. Heat a large saucepan over medium heat.
2. Add the oil.
3. Once the oil is hot, add the chicken breasts to the pan.
4. Brown the chicken on each side for 3-4 minutes, or until golden brown.
5. Remove the chicken from the pan and set it to one side.
6. Add the celery and carrot with a pinch of salt to the saucepan.
7. Stir the vegetables over the heat for 6 minutes.
8. Add the browned chicken back to the pan along with any juices from the meat.
9. Over the chicken and vegetables, add the tomatoes, stock, paste, oregano, garlic oil, parsley, and coconut sugar.
10. Mix well and cover.
11. Gently simmer for 20 minutes, or until the chicken is cooked through and the sauce is slightly thickened.
12. Meanwhile, boil the potatoes in a saucepan of boiling water for 10-12 minutes, or until tender and cooked through.
13. Drain the potatoes and serve alongside the chicken and tomatoes.

Per serving: Calories: 324 Protein: 35g Carbs: 21g Fiber: 5g Sugar: 6g Fat: 11g

Sautéed Herby Greek Chicken

SERVES 2 / PREP TIME: 10 MINUTES / COOK TIME: 25 MINUTES

Greek ingredients liven up your chicken!

---

2 tbsp olive oil
2 boneless, skinless chicken breasts
1 cup tomatoes, diced
1 tbsp balsamic vinegar
6 pimiento-stuffed green olives, thickly sliced
1 cup low FODMAP chicken stock
1 tbsp dried oregano
1 tsp dried parsley
1 tsp chopped green onion, green tips only
1 tbsp garlic-infused olive oil

---

1. Heat the oil in a large non-stick frying pan.
2. Sauté the chicken for 6-8 minutes.
3. Lift the chicken from the pan and set aside.
4. To the pan, add the tomatoes with the balsamic vinegar, olives, stock, herbs, green onions, and the garlic oil.
5. Now simmer, stirring frequently, for 7-8 minutes, or until pulpy.
6. Return the chicken and any juices to the pan and gently simmer, covered, for 5 minutes more, to finish cooking the chicken.
7. Serve hot.

Per serving: Calories: 387 Protein: 32g Carbs: 7g Fiber: 2g Sugar: 4g Fat: 26g

Red Pepper and Tomato Chicken

SERVES 2 / PREP TIME: 10 MINUTES / COOK TIME: 40 MINUTES

This easy baked chicken makes the perfect evening meal.

---

1 cup small red potatoes, thinly sliced
1 large zucchini, sliced
1 small yellow squash, sliced
1 red bell pepper, seeded and cubed
6 roma tomatoes, halved
A pinch of salt to taste
2 (5 oz) skinless boneless chicken breasts
3 tbsp olive oil

---

1. Preheat the oven to 400 degrees.
2. Spread the potatoes, zucchini, squash, pepper, and tomatoes in a glass baking dish.
3. Season this dish with the salt.
4. Meanwhile, score the flesh of each chicken breast 3-4 times using a sharp knife.
5. Lay the chicken on top of the vegetables.
6. Drizzle the olive oil over chicken.
7. Cover the dish with foil.
8. Bake for 30 minutes.
9. Remove the foil from the dish.
10. Return the dish to the oven.
11. Bake for 10 more minutes, or until the vegetables are juicy and the chicken is cooked through.

Hint: The juices from the chicken should run clear when pierced with a knife or toothpick.

Per serving: Calories: 318 Protein: 4g Carbs: 18g Fiber: 5gSugar: 5g Fat: 28g

Ginger Lime Chicken and Pumpkin

SERVES 2 / PREP TIME: 10 MINUTES / COOK TIME: 30 MINUTES

This refreshing pumpkin and lime dish makes a great Fall dinner!

---

1 lime, zest and juice
1 tbsp pure maple syrup
1 tsp grated fresh ginger
2 (5 oz) skinless, boneless chicken breasts
1 tbsp olive oil
1 tbsp fresh ginger, sliced into thin strips

2 cups fresh pumpkin purée
A pinch of salt and pepper to taste

---

1. Mix half the lime zest and all the lime juice with the maple syrup and grated ginger.
2. Score each chicken breast 3-4 times with a sharp knife.
3. Coat the breasts well with the marinade in a glass dish.
4. Set aside for 10 minutes so the chicken can marinate.
5. Meanwhile, preheat the broiler on low.
6. Line a baking tray with aluminum foil.
7. Place the marinated chicken breasts on the foil-lined tray.
8. Bake for 10-15 minutes under the broiler, flipping halfway through.
9. Bake until the chicken is cooked through and slightly caramelized.
10. While the chicken is baking, heat the oil in a small frying pan.
11. When the oil is hot, add the ginger strips.
12. Sauté them for 1 minute, or until the ginger is crisp.
13. Strain out the ginger with a slotted spoon, leaving the oil in the pan and placing ginger strips on a paper towel to one side.
14. Now stir the pumpkin purée into the ginger-infused oil.
15. Season the purée with the salt and pepper.
16. Sauté the purée until warmed through.
17. To serve, divide the pumpkin between 2 plates.
18. Top each plate with a chicken breast and the crisp ginger strips.

Hint: Green beans make a nice addition to this meal.

Per serving: Calories: 308 Protein: 33g Carbs: 21g Fiber: 3g Sugar: 10g Fat: 11g

Mexican Chicken and Pepper Tacos

SERVES 4 / PREP TIME: 5 MINUTES / COOK TIME: 45 MINUTES

This healthy taco recipe is sure to satisfy any taco craving!

---

1 (15 oz) can diced tomatoes
1 tbsp garlic-infused olive oil
1 large handful fresh cilantro leaves, chopped
1 tbsp olive oil
1 red bell pepper, de-seeded and thinly sliced
1 yellow bell pepper, de-seeded and thinly sliced

4 (5 oz) skinless chicken breasts, cut into thin strips
A pinch of paprika
A pinch of ground cumin
A pinch of dried oregano
A pinch of dried cilantro
4 gluten free tortillas
½ iceberg lettuce head, finely shredded

---

1. Preheat the oven to 350 degrees.
2. For the salsa, combine the tomatoes, garlic infused oil, and cilantro in a bowl.
3. Cover this bowl and chill for 30 minutes.
4. Heat the oil in a wok or large non-stick frying pan over medium-high heat.
5. Add the peppers.
6. Stir fry the peppers for 3-4 minutes.
7. Add the chicken strips, paprika, cumin, oregano, and cilantro.
8. Cook this for 10 minutes, or until the chicken is cooked through.
9. Meanwhile, wrap the tortillas in foil.
10. Warm them in the oven for 5 minutes.
11. Spoon one-quarter of the chicken mixture into the center of each tortilla.
12. Add a little salsa and shredded lettuce to each tortilla.
13. Roll up and serve warm.

Per serving: Calories: 328 Protein: 35g Carbs: 22g Fiber: 6g Sugar: 6g Fat: 12g

Roasted Moroccan Spiced Chicken

SERVES 8 / PREP TIME: 20 MINUTES / COOK TIME: 40 MINUTES

This spiced chicken recipe is perfect for a dinner party!

---

2 lemons
2 tsp ground turmeric
2 tsp ground cumin
2 tbsp olive oil
A pinch of salt and pepper to taste
8 (5 oz) skinless chicken breasts
4 red potatoes
1/2 tsp turmeric

---

1. Preheat the oven to 425 degrees.
2. Finely grate the zest from 1 lemon.
3. Squeeze the juice from both the lemons into a large, shallow dish.
4. Toss in the turmeric, cumin, half the oil, and some salt and pepper.
5. Add the chicken breasts to the dish.
6. Cover the dish and marinate for as long as possible in the fridge.
7. Meanwhile, cut the potatoes in half.
8. Spread them over the bottom of a roasting dish.
9. Toss the potatoes in the remaining oil.
10. Sprinkle the potatoes with the turmeric.
11. Set the chicken on a rack above the potatoes in the oven.
12. Bake both dishes at the same time for 30-40 minutes, or until the chicken is well browned and the potatoes are tender.

Per serving: Calories: 227 Protein: 32g Carbs: 8g Fiber: 1g Sugar: 1g Fat: 7g

North African Baked Chicken

SERVES 4 / PREP TIME: 10 MINUTES / COOK TIME: 50 MINUTES

The delicious spices of Northern Africa shine in this simple baked dish.

---

2 white potatoes, peeled and cut into 1 inch cubes
2 carrots, peeled and cut into 1 inch cubes
2 tbsp garlic-infused olive oil
A pinch of salt to taste

4 (5 oz) chicken breasts
1 lemon, quartered
1 tsp ground cumin
1 tsp turmeric

---

1. Preheat the oven to 400 degrees.
2. Place the potatoes and carrots into a roasting dish.
3. Drizzle the oil over the vegetables.
4. Season them well with salt.
5. Place the dish in the oven to roast for 30 minutes.
6. Once roasted, remove the dish from the oven.
7. Add the chicken breasts and lemon quarters in a single layer over the vegetables.
8. Sprinkle everything with the spices.
9. Roast the chicken for 15-20 more minutes, or until the chicken is cooked through.
10. To serve, divide the chicken among four plates, each with a slice of roasted lemon for squeezing over the food.

Per serving: Calories: 389 Protein: 34g Carbs: 25g Fiber: 4g Sugar: 3g Fat: 17g

Homemade Tomato and Turkey Gnocchi

SERVES 4 / PREP TIME: 30 MINUTES / COOK TIME: 10 MINUTES

This delicious homemade gnocchi recipe is perfect for a cold winter evening!

---

4 white potatoes, washed and peeled
1/2 cup brown rice flour
1 cup white rice flour
1/4 cup sorghum flour
1/4 cup tapioca flour
1 cup potato starch

2 egg whites, lightly beaten
A pinch of salt to taste
Water for boiling the gnocchi
1 tbsp garlic infused oil
1 cup tomatoes, diced
1 tbsp dried oregano
4 (5 oz) turkey breasts, cooked and sliced

---

1. Slice the potatoes.
2. Steam over high heat for about 10 minutes, or until tender.
3. Place the potatoes in a food processor and process until smooth.
4. Meanwhile, mix all the flours and the potato starch together by sifting through a mesh strainer into a mixing bowl.
5. Scrape the blended potato into this bowl.
6. Now add the lightly beaten egg whites.
7. Season this mixture with the salt.
8. Stir this mixture together until it forms a dough.
9. Turn out the dough onto a lightly floured surface.
10. Form it into a ball.
11. Cut the dough ball into four sections.
12. Roll out each section into a long cylinder about 4 inches wide.
13. Cut each cylinder into 1 inch pieces.
14. Meanwhile, boil a medium pan of water (about 3/4 full).
15. Add half the gnocchi to the water for approximately 3 minutes.
16. When the gnocchi float to the top of the water, they are done.
17. Scoop them out with a slotted spoon and add to a serving bowl.
18. Repeat with the rest of the gnocchi.
19. Now heat the garlic-infused oil in a skillet over medium heat.
20. Add the diced tomatoes and oregano to the hot oil.
21. Add in the cooked turkey slices.
22. Allow this mixture to warm thoroughly, about 3 minutes.
23. Pour the tomatoes and turkey over the gnocchi in the serving bowl and tuck in!

Per serving: Calories: 750 Protein: 54g Carbs: 121g Sugar: 3g Fat: 7g

Crock Pot Turkey Stuffed Peppers

SERVES 4 / PREP TIME: 10 MINUTES / COOK TIME: 3-4 HOURS

These savory stuffed peppers can be cooking while you're at work!

---

4 large bell peppers, a mix of colors
1 lb ground turkey
1 tbsp chopped fresh rosemary
1 tbsp chopped fresh oregano
1 medium stalk celery, chopped
1 tbsp garlic infused oil
2 cups cooked brown rice
2 cups diced tomatoes
1 cup feta cheese, crumbled
A pinch of salt to taste
1 tbsp chives (green tips only), thinly
sliced

---

1. Cut the tops off the bell peppers and remove the seeds.
2. In a medium bowl, mix the ground turkey, rosemary, oregano, celery, garlic oil, rice, 1 cup the diced tomatoes, half the feta cheese, and a pinch of salt to taste.
3. Spoon equal amounts of the meat mixture into the bell peppers.
4. Place the rest of the diced tomatoes into the bottom of the crock pot.
5. Add the peppers to the crock pot on top of the tomatoes, keeping the peppers sitting upright.
6. Turn the crock pot on high for 3-4 hours (or 7 hours on low).
7. 5 minutes before serving, sprinkle the remaining cheese on top of the cooked bell peppers.
8. Then top with the sliced chives.
9. To serve, drizzle the tomato sauce from the bottom of the crock pot on top of each pepper.

Per serving: Calories: 419 Protein: 35g Carbs: 37g Fiber: 6g Sugar: 8g Fat: 1g

Pan Fried Cilantro Cajun Chicken

SERVES 4 / PREP TIME: 10 MINUTES / COOK TIME: 20 MINUTES

Spicy and fresh flavors.

For the salsa:
¼ cup fresh cilantro, chopped roughly
2 green onions (green tips) only, chopped
3 tomatoes, diced
1 lime
1 tbsp olive oil
A pinch of salt and pepper to taste

For the chicken:
1 tsp dried oregano
2 tsp ground cumin
2 tsp ground cilantro seeds
2 tsp smoked paprika
½ tsp salt
4 (5 oz) skinless chicken breasts
1 tbsp olive oil

---

1. Mix the ingredients for the salsa in a serving bowl.
2. Meanwhile, mix the oregano, and spices together in a shallow bowl.
3. Coat the chicken in this mixture.
4. Cover the chicken with parchment paper.
5. Beat the chicken with a rolling pin or meat mallet to flatten it out.
6. Now place the chicken in a pan with the oil over medium heat.
7. Cook the chicken for 15-20 minutes, turning half way through, until it is golden and cooked through.
8. Slice up the chicken and serve with salsa on the side.

Per serving: Calories: 267 Protein: 33g Carbs: 9g Fiber: 3g Sugar: 4g Fat: 11g

Oriental Sweet and Sour Chicken

SERVES 3 / PREP TIME: 5 MINUTES / COOK TIME: 25 MINUTES

Delicious!

---

9 tbsp tomato paste
1 (20 oz) can pineapple chunks, drained
2 red bell peppers, seeded and cut into chunks
3 tbsp rice wine vinegar
4 tbsp stevia/coconut sugar
1 tbsp coconut oil
4 (5 oz) skinless and boneless chicken breast, sliced

1 cup cooked brown rice
1 green onions, sliced (green tips only)

---

1. In a large bowl, combine the tomato paste, pineapple, bell peppers, vinegar, and stevia/sugar.
2. Next, heat the oil in a skillet over medium-high heat.
3. Sauté the chicken breasts for 6-7 minutes before turning.
4. Sauté for 2-3 more minutes after turning them over.
5. Now add the tomato sauce to the skillet.
6. Cover the skillet and let it simmer for 15 minutes, or until the chicken is thoroughly cooked.
7. Serve with cooked rice and a sprinkle of green onions.

Per serving: Calories: 502 Protein: 46g Carbs: 56g Fiber: 7g Sugar: 35g Fat: 1g

Chilled Thai Chicken Salad

SERVES 2 / PREP TIME: 30 MINUTES / COOK TIME: NA

A delicious cold and crisp Thai-infused chicken salad dish.

---

3 limes, juiced
1 tbsp fish sauce
1 tbsp coconut sugar
2 (4 oz) cooked skinless chicken breasts, shredded
½ cucumber, cut into strips
1 tbsp chopped chives
1 tbsp fresh mint leaves

1 tbsp fresh cilantro leaves
½ cup bean sprouts, cooked

---

1. To make the marinade, mix the lime juice, fish sauce, and sugar together until the sugar dissolves.
2. Add the rest of the ingredients to a salad bowl.
3. Drizzle the salad with the marinade.
4. Cover and refrigerate until completely chilled (or at least 30 minutes).
5. Serve chilled.

Per serving: Calories: 188 Protein: 28g Carbs: 12g Fiber: 2g Sugar: 5g Fat: 4g

Chicken Tagine

SERVES 2 / PREP TIME: 5 MINUTES / COOK TIME: 3.5-4 HOURS SLOW COOKER

A Northern African inspired dish.

---

2 carrots, peeled and sliced
2 (4oz) chicken breasts, skinless and boneless, diced
1 cup low FODMAP chicken stock
2 tbsp rice flour
2 tbsp lemon juice, freshly squeezed
1 ½ tsp ground cumin
1 ½ tsp ground ginger

1 tsp ground nutmeg
¾ tsp ground black pepper
1 cup water
2 cups cooked white rice
3 tbsp fresh cilantro, finely chopped

---

1. Add the carrots and chicken into the slow cooker.
2. In a bowl, whisk the stock, flour, lemon juice, cumin, ginger, nutmeg and the ground black pepper.
3. Add the mixture to the cooker along with the water.
4. Cover and cook on low for 6 ½ to 7 hours or on High for 3 ½ to 4 hours.
5. Serve the rice in bowls and ladle over the tagine.
6. Garnish with cilantro to finish.

Per serving: Calories: 215 Protein: 35g Carbs: 7g Fiber: 1g Sugar: 1g Fat: 5g

Chicken and Lemon Rice Stew

SERVES 3 / PREP TIME: 15 MINUTES / COOK TIME: 6-7 HOURS SLOW COOKER

Chicken and lemon pairs fantastically in this simple dish.

1 tbsp olive oil
2 (4 oz) chicken breasts, skinless and boneless, diced
1/2 cup celery, chopped
1/3 cup carrot, chopped
1 cup low FODMAP chicken stock
1 cup water
1 tsp dried oregano

A pinch of black pepper
1 cup white rice, rinsed and drained
1 lemon, juiced
1/2 cucumber, washed and sliced
1 cup spinach, washed
1 tbsp extra virgin olive oil

1. Heat the oil in a skillet over medium heat.
2. Add the chicken breasts.
3. Cook for 3-5 minutes, stirring often until browned.
4. Stir in the celery and carrot.
5. Cook for 2 minutes, stirring occasionally.
6. Drain off the excess juices.
7. Into the slow cooker, add the chicken mixture and remaining ingredients (except lemon, extra virgin olive oil, cucumber and spinach).
8. Cover with the lid and cook on high for 30 minutes.
9. Reduce the heat to low.
10. Cook for 6-7 hours on low, or until the rice is tender and the liquid is absorbed.
11. Stir in the juice of half a lemon.
12. Slice the cucumber and mix with the spinach for the side salad.
13. Whisk the remaining lemon juice and olive oil together.
14. Dress the salad with the lemon and oil dressing.
15. Serve on the side of your chicken.

Per serving: Calories: 450 Protein: 29g Carbs: 54g Fiber: 2g Sugar: 0g Fat: 13g

Slow-Cooked Chicken Masala

SERVES 3 / PREP TIME: 15 MINUTES / COOK TIME: 4.5 HOURS SLOW COOKER

The fragrant spices release in the slow cooker, giving this dish an authentic taste.

---

2 (4 oz) skinless, boneless chicken breasts, diced
1/2 red bell pepper, chopped
1/2 yellow bell pepper, chopped
1/2 cup green onions (green tips only), sliced
1 cup low FODMAP chicken stock
1 tbsp mild curry powder

1/4 tsp turmeric
1/2 cup almond milk
1 tsp cornstarch (or potato starch)
1 cup white rice, cooked
2 tbsp fresh cilantro, chopped

---

1. Combine the chicken, peppers, green onions, stock, curry powder and turmeric in the slow cooker.
2. Cover and cook on low for 8- 9 hours or on high for 4½ hours.
3. In a small bowl, mix the almond milk and cornstarch until smooth.
4. Stir into the chicken mixture.
5. If you're cooking on low, turn up the heat to high now.
6. Cover and cook for 15 to 20 minutes more.
7. The sauce should be slightly thickened by now.
8. Serve on white rice and sprinkle with cilantro to finish.

Per serving: Calories: 259 Protein: 27g Carbs: 26g Fiber: 2g Sugar: 5g Fat: 5g

Fennel and Ginger Chicken

SERVES 4 / PREP TIME: 5 MINUTES / COOK TIME: 2.5-3 HOURS SLOW COOKER

The bold flavors of fennel, ginger and garlic are delicious.

---

3 (4 oz) skinless boneless chicken breasts, diced
1/4 tsp ground black pepper
1 bulb fennel, cored and cut into thin wedges
1 red bell pepper, de-seeded and diced
1 tsp fresh or dried rosemary
1 tsp fresh or dried ginger (finely sliced

if fresh)
½ cup low FODMAP chicken stock
1 cup water
1 tbsp dried oregano

---

1. Sprinkle the chicken pieces with ground pepper.
2. Place the chicken into the slow cooker.
3. Top with fennel, bell pepper, rosemary and ginger.
4. Add the stock and water.
5. Cover and cook on low for 5 to 6 hours or on high for 2½ to 3 hours.
6. Sprinkle each serving with oregano to finish.

Per serving: Calories: 166 Protein: 27g Carbs: 6g Fiber: 2g Sugar: 3g Fat: 4g

Rich Tomato and Red Pepper Chicken

SERVES 4 / PREP TIME: 5 MINUTES / COOK TIME: 3.5-4 HOURS SLOW COOKER

A tasty comforting slow cooked stew.

---

12 oz skinless, boneless chicken thighs, cut into cubes
½ tsp dried oregano
¼ tsp ground black pepper
1 cup low FODMAP chicken stock
1 cup water
1 medium red bell pepper, roughly chopped

1 cup sliced large tomatoes
1 tsp cumin
1 cup cooked white rice

---

1. Into the slow cooker, combine the chicken, oregano and black pepper.
2. Add in the stock and water.
3. Cover and cook on low for 7 to 8 hours or on high for 3 ½ to 4 hours.
4. If using low, turn the heat up to high after 3.5-4 hours.
5. Stir in the red pepper, tomatoes and cumin.
6. Cover and cook for another 30 minutes.
7. Serve steaming hot with fluffy white rice.

Per serving: Calories: 179 Protein: 15g Carbs: 21g Fiber: 1g Sugar: 5g Fat: 4g

Caribbean Style Chicken Thighs

SERVES 2 / PREP TIME: 5 MINUTES / COOK TIME: 7-8 HOURS SLOW COOKER

Slowly infusing the spices into this Caribbean dish ensures an authentic taste.

---

1 tsp cumin
1 tsp cinnamon
1 tsp dried oregano
1 tbsp garlic-infused olive oil
8 oz chicken thighs, skinless and boneless
A pinch of black pepper
1 lime, juice
2 tbsp fresh cilantro, chopped

---

1. Mix the dry spices, herbs and garlic oil in a bowl to form your marinade.
2. Marinate the chicken thighs in the spice mix for as long as you've got!
3. Place in the bottom of the slow cooker in a single layer.
4. Cook for 7-8 hours on a low setting.
5. Remove the turkey thighs from the slow cooker.
6. Place them onto a chopping board.
7. Cut the thighs into slices.
8. Squeeze over the fresh lime juice and scatter over the fresh cilantro to serve.

Per serving: Calories: 272 Protein: 28g Carbs: 5g Fiber: 2g Sugar: 1g Fat: 16g

VEGETARIAN

Slow Cooked Autumn Root Vegetables

SERVES 6 / PREP TIME: 10 MINUTES / COOK TIME: 3-4 HOURS SLOW COOKER

Satisfying root vegetables slow cooked to perfection.

---

1 cup boiling water
1 tbsp rice flour
1 small rutabaga, peeled and cubed
2 large carrots, peeled and cubed
2 turnips, peeled and cubed
1 cup low FODMAP vegetable stock
2 tbsp dried oregano
Freshly ground black pepper, to taste

---

1. Dissolve the flour in the boiling water and transfer to the slow cooker pot.
2. Add all of the remaining ingredients to the slow cooker.
3. Set the slow cooker to low for 3-4 hours until cooked through.

Per serving: Calories: 35 Protein: 2g Carbs: 7g Fiber: 2g Sugar: 3g Fat: 0g

Greek Rice

SERVES 6/ PREP TIME: 10 MINUTES / COOK TIME: 2 HOURS SLOW COOKER

Rice can be a pain to cook, but not with this recipe. The Greek flavors add an extra touch.

---

1 tbsp garlic-infused olive oil
2 cups white rice
3 cups water
1 cup low FODMAP vegetable stock
1 red bell pepper, seeds and pith re-moved, and finely chopped
1 green bell pepper, seeds and pith re-moved, and finely chopped

1 cup crumbled feta cheese
2 tbsp lemon juice

---

1. Heat the oil in a deep frying pan over medium heat.
2. Add the rice and sauté until the rice is nicely browned.
3. Transfer to the slow cooker pot.
4. Add the water and stock to the pan, and de-glaze the frying pan.
5. Transfer to the slow cooker.
6. Set the slow cooker to high for 2 hours.
7. With 30 minutes left of the cooking time, fluff the rice, and mix in the bell pepper and cheese.
8. When the rice is cooked to your desired consistency, stir in the lemon juice.

Per serving: Calories: 332 Protein: 9g Carbs: 54g Fiber: 1g Sugar: 3g Fat: 8g

Roasted Eggplant

SERVES 2 / PREP TIME: 10 MINUTES / COOK TIME: 40 MINUTES

Delicious Middle Eastern Flavors.

---

4 cups eggplant (approx. 1 medium eggplant, diced)
A pinch of salt
2 tbsp garlic-infused olive oil
1 tbsp dried oregano
1 tbsp fresh basil leaves, torn
1 lemon, juice

---

1. Preheat the oven to 300 degrees.
2. Slice the eggplant in half lengthways.
3. Use the knife to lightly score across the flesh in crosses.
4. Sprinkle with salt and leave for a few minutes.
5. Line a baking sheet with parchment paper.
6. Place the eggplant on the sheet(skin side down).
7. Drizzle over the oil and oregano.
8. Roast in the oven for 30-40 minutes or until very soft.
9. Serve with the fresh basil and a squeeze of lemon juice.

Per serving: Calories: 191 Protein: 2g Carbs: 18g Fiber: 5g Sugar: 6g Fat: 14g

Mixed Vegetable Minestrone Soup

SERVES 5 / PREP TIME: 5 MINUTES / COOK TIME: 40 MINUTES

A classic!

---

2 tbsp olive oil
1 celery stalk, sliced
2 medium carrots, peeled and diced
2 medium potatoes, peeled and diced
2 medium zucchinis, peeled and diced
2 cups low FODMAP vegetable stock
1 cup beef tomatoes, diced
½ tsp dried parsley

½ tsp dried basil
A pinch of salt and pepper
1 1/2 cups gluten free macaroni pasta

---

1. In a large soup pot, heat the olive oil and sauté the celery and carrot until soft.
2. Add the carrots, potatoes, zucchinis, vegetable stock, tomatoes, herbs, salt, and pepper.
3. Bring to a rolling boil.
4. Lower the heat slightly and allow to simmer for 20 minutes.
5. Add the gluten free macaroni to the pot.
6. Simmer for 15 minutes until the pasta is thoroughly cooked.
7. Serve hot.

Per serving: Calories: 274 Protein: 8g Carbs: 46g Fiber: 5g Sugar: 0g Fat: 7g

Gluten Free Tomato and Basil Pasta

SERVES 2 / PREP TIME: 5 MINUTES / COOK TIME: 15 MINUTES

Ready in a flash!

---

1 ½ cup gluten free penne pasta (or
equivalent shape)
½ cup beef tomatoes, finely diced and
juices reserved
1 tbsp garlic-infused olive oil
1 lemon, juice
A pinch of salt and pepper
1 tbsp fresh basil, torn

---

1.   Cook pasta according to package directions.
2.   Drain and allow to cool.
3.   Mix through the tomatoes, oil, lemon juice and salt and pepper.
4.   Top with torn basil and serve!

Per serving: Calories: 426 Protein: 14g Carbs: 73g Fiber: 6g Sugar: 4g Fat: 9g

Herby Carrot and Lemon Soup

SERVES 4 /   PREP TIME:15 MINUTES /   COOK TIME: 7-8 HOURS SLOW COOKER

This soup is amazing and fresh.

1 tbsp olive oil
1 tsp fennel seeds, crushed
1 tbsp ground ginger
4 medium carrots, peeled and chopped
1 cup green onions (green tips only), diced
1 lemon, zest and juice

4 cups water
2 tbsp fresh oregano, chopped
Freshly ground black pepper, to taste

1. Heat the oil in a skillet over medium heat.
2. Add the crushed fennel seeds and stir-fry for a minute.
3. Add the ground ginger and cook for another minute.
4. Add the carrots, green onions, and lemon juice and cook until the vegetables are softened, about 5 minutes.
5. Remove from the heat and transfer to the slow cooker pot.
6. Add the water, lemon zest, and fresh oregano to the pot.
7. Season generously with freshly ground black pepper.
8. Set the slow cooker to LOW for 7-8 hours overnight.
9. Blend in a food processor for a smooth soup if desired or simply ladle straight from the slow cooker for a chunkier stock.

Per serving: Calories: 66 Protein: 1g Carbs: 9g Fiber: 3g Sugar: 3g Fat: 4g

Veggie Quinoa and Parsley Burgers

SERVES 4 / PREP TIME: 10 MINUTES / COOK TIME: 15 MINUTES

Packed with protein and succulent flavors – you won't miss the meat!

1 tsp ground cumin
1 medium zucchini, diced
3/4 cup quinoa, cooked
1 medium carrot, peeled and grated
1 stalk celery, sliced
1 tbsp dried parsley
A pinch of salt and pepper
2 egg whites
1 tbsp quinoa flour

1 tbsp olive oil
1 cup organic spinach, washed

1. Add all of the ingredients (except oil and spinach) into a mixing bowl and stir well.
2. Then, add your egg and quinoa flour and stir.
3. Form between 4 veggie patties and dust with a little extra quinoa powder.
4. Place the veggie patties on a covered plate or in a container and set aside in the refrigerator to cool for at least either an hour or overnight.
5. In a skillet, heat the olive oil and cook the patties for 6-7 minutes on each side or until golden brown on the outside and piping hot in the middle.
6. Serve with the freshly washed spinach on the side.

Per serving: Calories: 191 Protein: 8g Carbs: 28g Fiber: 5g Sugar: 3g Fat: 6g

Roasted Tomato and Basil Soup

SERVES 5 / PREP TIME: 10 MINUTES / COOK TIME: 50 MINUTES

Roasting your tomatoes adds a real sweet kick to a traditional tomato soup.

---

5 beef tomatoes, halved
1 tbsp olive oil
A pinch of salt and pepper
2 cups low FODMAP vegetable stock
1 cup water
1/2 cup + 1 tbsp fresh basil, torn

---

1. Preheat the oven to 300 degrees.
2. Add the tomatoes to a parchment-lined baking sheet.
3. Then, drizzle the oil over the tomatoes and sprinkle with salt and pepper.
4. Roast the tomatoes for 20-30 minutes until lightly browned.
5. Then, into a large saucepan over medium heat, add the roasted tomatoes, , stock, water, and 1/2 cup basil.
6. Bring to a gentle boil and then lower the heat to simmer for 20 minutes.
7. Remove and allow to cool slightly before blending with a stick blender or in a processor.
8. Scatter the extra torn basil over the top and serve.

Per Serving: Calories: 34 Protein: 2 g Carbs: 7g Fiber: 2g Sugar: 4g Fat: 0g

Spinach, Carrot and Quinoa Salad

SERVES 4 / PREP TIME: 5 MINUTES / COOK TIME: 20 MINUTES

A refreshing vegan salad.

---

1 cup quinoa
1 tbsp olive oil
½ tsp cumin
½ tsp paprika
1 1/3 cups water
2 cups organic spinach, washed
1 carrot, peeled and grated
2 beef tomatoes, washed and sliced
1 tbsp fresh chives (green tips only),
chopped
1 lime, juice and zest
A pinch of salt and pepper

---

1. First, rinse the quinoa thoroughly in cold water.
2. Drain the quinoa and set aside.
3. Use a medium saucepan to heat up the oil over medium heat.
4. Then, add the spices, stirring for 30 seconds.
5. Add the quinoa to the pan and stir.
6. Continue cooking for 2 minutes whilst stirring.
7. Now add the water and turn down to a simmer for 15 minutes or until the water has mostly been absorbed.
8. Spread the quinoa over the bottom of a shallow bowl and allow it to cool down to room temperature.
9. Mix the cooked quinoa with the spinach, carrots, tomatoes, and chives.
10. Squeeze the lime juice onto the salad and scatter over the lime zest - toss to coat.
11. Season with salt and pepper to serve.

Per Serving: Calories: 205 Protein: 7g Carbs: 32g Fiber: 5g Sugar: 3g Fat: 6g

Mason Jar Pineapple and Rice Salad

SERVES 2 / PREP TIME: 5 MINUTES / COOK TIME: 20 MINUTES

Deliciously sweet!

---

1 cup red jasmine rice
1 tsp olive oil
1 tsp white wine vinegar
A pinch of salt and pepper
2 cups organic spinach, washed
1 cup canned pineapple chunks
1 tbsp freshly chopped mint

2 glass mason jars

---

1. Cook the rice according to package directions.
2. Whisk the oil, vinegar, salt and pepper together to form your dressing.
3. Into the mason jars, layer half the cooked rice followed with spinach, then pineapple chunks.
4. Press down and repeat until the jar is almost full.
5. Repeat for the second jar.
6. When ready to eat, pour over a little dressing, place the lid on securely, give it a little shake and enjoy!

Per Serving: Calories: 176, Protein: 4g , Carbs: 35g , Fiber: 3g, Sugar: 10g, Fat: 3g

Potato and Scallion Soup

SERVES 5 / PREP TIME: 10 MINUTES / COOK TIME: 30 MINUTES

Wholesome and fresh.

---

2 cups low FODMAP vegetable stock
1 cup rice milk
5 small white potatoes, peeled and diced
2 tbsp chives, chopped
2 carrots, peeled and diced

¼ cup scallions (green tips only), sliced
1 tbsp olive oil
1 tbsp dried parsley
1 tsp dried rosemary
A pinch of sea salt

---

1. Into a large stock pot, add the vegetable stock, milk, potatoes, chives, carrots and scallions and bring to a boil over high heat.
2. Next, add in the olive oil, parsley, rosemary, and salt.
3. Lower the heat and allow the mixture to simmer for 30 minutes until the potatoes are tender, whilst occasionally stirring to prevent the bottom from sticking – if it starts to dry out simply add a little water/milk.
4. Allow to cool slightly and blend until smooth.
5. Serve hot!

Per Serving: Calories: 102, Protein: 2g, Carbs: 16g, Fiber: 2g, Sugar: 5g, Fat: 3g

Pumpkin and Tomato Vegetable Soup

SERVES 4 / PREP TIME: 5 MINUTES / COOK TIME: 1 HOUR AND 15 MINUTES

This savory soup makes the perfect dinner treat!

---

1 tbsp garlic-infused olive oil
3 tomatoes, coarsely chopped
1 cup water
1 bundle of herbs tied with a string: 1 bay leaf, 2 thyme sprigs, and 1 rosemary sprig
A pinch of salt
2 medium carrots, diced
1 turnip, diced

1 (15 oz) cup pumpkin purée
1 cup water
1 cup fresh or frozen spinach
1 cup quinoa
1 tsp dried oregano

---

1. Heat the olive oil in a large, deep pan over medium-high heat.
2. Reduce the heat to medium.
3. Add the tomatoes and let them cook for 15 minutes, or until thickened.
4. Add the water and the bundle of herbs.
5. Bring the water to a boil.
6. Sprinkle the water with the salt.
7. Now add the carrots, turnip and pumpkin.
8. Reduce the heat to minimum.
9. Simmer for 40 minutes, or until the vegetables are slightly tender.
10. Next add another cup water, the spinach, and the quinoa and cook over medium-low heat for 20 minutes.
11. Remove the bundle of herbs.
12. Sprinkle the oregano over the soup.
13. Ladle it into bowls to serve.

Per serving: Calories: 319 Protein: 8g Carbs: 45g Fiber: 9g Sugar: 10g Fat: 13g

Carrot and Cucumber Spring Rolls

SERVES 2 / PREP TIME: 20 MINUTES / COOK TIME: 10 MINUTES

This nearly no-cook method will give you restaurant-quality spring rolls in no time!

---

2 medium carrots, peeled
1/2 cucumber
1 medium zucchini, peeled and sliced
1 tbsp fresh cilantro, chopped
1 tsp low sodium soy sauce
1 tsp rice wine vinegar
1/2 tsp sesame oil
2 oz water to boil the noodles
1 oz rice noodles

10 spring roll wrappers
1/2 tsp sesame oil
1 tsp rice wine vinegar
1 tsp fresh cilantro, chopped

---

1. Julienne the carrots, cucumber, and zucchini, keeping each vegetable separate.
2. Make the dressing for the carrots by mixing the cilantro, soy sauce, rice wine vinegar, and sesame oil.
3. Drizzle this over the julienned carrots in a small bowl.
4. Meanwhile, in large saucepan, boil the water in preparation for the rice noodles.
5. Cook them according to package directions.
6. Drain the noodles and set them aside.
7. Hydrate the spring roll wrappers by adding then individually to a large bowl filled with very warm water.
8. Remove them from the water when they are fully pliable.
9. Place them onto a plastic cutting board.
10. Place the noodles and veggies near the edge of each wrapper.
11. Roll them up burrito-style.
12. Meanwhile, create a light dipping sauce with sesame oil, rice wine vinegar, and a sprinkling of cilantro to taste.
13. Cut the spring rolls diagonally and enjoy.

Hint: To julienne the vegetables, slice primarily the outer skin, not the center.

Per serving: Calories: 277, Protein: 6g Carbs: 58g, Sugar: 5g, Fat: 3g

Quinoa and Carrot Salad with Lemon Cilantro Dressing

SERVES 3 / PREP TIME: 5 MINUTES / COOK TIME: 20 MINUTES

This filling salad can be an entire meal by itself!

1 cup red quinoa
1/4 cup garlic-infused olive oil
1/2 tbsp fresh lemon juice
1 cup fresh cilantro leaves, washed
A pinch of salt to taste
2 small carrots, peeled and sliced
1 small zucchini, peeled and sliced
1/4 cup black olives, sliced

1/2 cup roma tomatoes, cut into wedges
2 cups fresh spinach, washed
3/4 cup canned chickpeas
1 yellow bell pepper, de-seeded and thinly sliced

1. Cook the quinoa by rinsing thoroughly with cold water.
2. Add to a pan of boiling water (2 cups).
3. Simmer with the lid on for 20 minutes.
4. Turn off the heat and allow to steam with the lid on whilst you prepare the rest of the salad.
5. Whisk together the garlic infused oil, fresh lemon juice, cilantro leaves, salt, and set aside.
6. Into a serving bowl, add the cooked quinoa.
7. Top the quinoa with the rest of the ingredients and the dressing and toss to coat.
8. Serve by scooping the salad into individual bowls.

Per serving: Calories: 368 Protein: 9g Carbs: 37g Fiber: 8g Sugar: 6g Fat: 22g

Zucchini and Carrot Spaghetti

SERVES 2 / PREP TIME: 5 MINUTES / COOK TIME: 15 MINUTES

This fun recipe transforms spaghetti into a gluten-free, low carb masterpiece.

2 medium zucchinis
1 tbsp garlic infused oil
2 large tomatoes, diced
2 medium carrots, peeled
1 small poblano pepper, de-seeded and sliced

A pinch of salt and pepper to taste
1 tbsp olive oil

1. Julienne the zucchinis (avoid the very soft center) and set aside.
2. In a large skillet, add the garlic infused oil, tomatoes, carrots, and pepper.
3. Sauté for 3 minutes.
4. Add in the zucchini.
5. Stir and cook until the veggies are fork tender, approx. 10 minutes.
6. Season with the salt and pepper.
7. Drizzle the spaghetti with olive oil to serve.

Per serving: Calories: 206 Protein: 4g Carbs: 18g Fiber: 6g Sugar: 12g Fat: 15g

Spinach and Feta Fusilli

SERVES 2 / PREP TIME: 10 MINUTES / COOK TIME: 15 MINUTES

This fast gluten free pasta recipe might surprise you with how flavorful it is.

---

7 oz gluten free fusilli
1 tbsp garlic-infused olive oil
2 cups fresh or frozen spinach, washed and drained
1 tsp crushed red pepper flakes
2 tbsp feta cheese, crumbled

A pinch of salt to taste
2 tbsp fresh basil, torn

---

1. Cook the fusilli according to package instructions.
2. Drain and set it aside.
3. Next, heat the oil in a skillet over medium-high heat.
4. Add the spinach.
5. Sauté for 5 minutes, or until wilted.
6. Add the cooked pasta, red pepper flakes, and feta cheese to the skillet.
7. Quickly give everything a stir.
8. Season generously with the salt, and basil.
9. Toss well and serve.

Per serving: Calories: 224 Protein: 7g Carbs: 27g Sugar: 3g Fat: 12g

Red Quinoa and Pumpkin Stew

SERVES 2 / PREP TIME: 15 MINUTES / COOK TIME: 1 HOUR AND 15 MINUTES

Deliciously chunky, herby soup.

---

3 tbsp garlic-infused olive oil
1 stalk celery, diced
3 large tomatoes, coarsely chopped
1 cup water
A bundle of herbs tied with a string: 1 bay leaf, 2 fresh thyme sprigs, and 1 fresh rosemary sprig

A pinch of salt
2 medium carrots, diced
1 turnip, diced
1 cup fresh cooked pumpkin, diced
1 cup water
1 cup fresh spinach
1 cup red quinoa

---

1. Heat the olive oil in a large deep pan over medium heat.
2. Add the celery and the tomatoes.
3. Let them cook for 15 minutes, or until thickened.
4. Add the water and the bundle of herbs.
5. Bring this to a boil.
6. Sprinkle in the salt and add the carrots, turnip, and pumpkin.
7. Reduce the heat to low.
8. Simmer the stew like this for 40 minutes, or until the vegetables are tender yet crisp.
9. Next, add the other cup water, the spinach, and the red quinoa.
10. Cook this over medium-low heat for about 20 minutes.
11. Remove the bundle of herbs before serving.

Per serving: Calories: 606 Protein: 16g Carbs: 81g Fiber: 15g Sugar: 16g Fat: 26g

Healthy Potatoes Dauphinoise

SERVES 4 / PREP TIME: 10 MINUTES / COOK TIME: 1 HOUR

This one-dish gourmet meal is sure to impress guests!

---

4 small white potatoes, sliced thinly
1 cup fresh cooked pumpkin, sliced thinly
1 tbsp coconut oil
2 tbsp potato starch

1 cup canned coconut milk
1 ½ tsp salt
1 tbsp fresh thyme, leaves only

---

1. Preheat the oven to 350 degrees.
2. Start layering the thinly sliced potatoes and pumpkin in a 9x13 baking dish.
3. Set this aside.
4. Use a medium saucepan to heat the coconut oil over medium-low heat until melted.
5. Add the potato starch.
6. Stir until the potato starch is smooth.
7. Allow it to simmer until the mixture turns light golden, about 5 minutes.
8. Meanwhile, heat the milk in a small saucepan.
9. Gradually add the warm milk to the potato starch by whisking continuously until smooth.
10. Bring this to a boil.
11. Cook for 10 minutes, stirring constantly.
12. Remove this from the heat.
13. Season with the salt.
14. Pour over the potatoes and pumpkin.
15. Transfer the baking dish to the oven.
16. Bake for 45 minutes until golden on top - finish under the broiler for a crispy topping.
17. Top the dish with fresh thyme to serve.

Hint: Use light coconut milk to reduce the amount of saturated fat content.

Per serving: Calories: 361 Protein: 6g Carbs: 48g Fiber: 7g Sugar: 4g Fat: 18g

Zucchini Citrus Veggie Fritters

SERVES 4 / PREP TIME: 10 MINUTES / COOK TIME: 30 MINUTES

Crunchy, succulent and mouthwatering.

½ cup quinoa
1 cup boiling water
A pinch of salt
4 tbsp olive oil
2 cups zucchini, diced
1/2 cup millet
½ cup chopped fresh parsley
¼ cup chives (green tops only), chopped

½ lemon, zest only
2 tbsp lemon juice
½ cup canned chickpeas
½ tsp salt
½ tsp cumin
2 egg whites
2 tbsp rice flour
1 tsp coconut oil

---

1. Rinse the quinoa under cold water.
1. Place the quinoa in a saucepan with the boiling water and the salt and simmer on medium heat for 20 minutes.
2. When the water is absorbed, stir with a fork to fluff and set aside.
3. In the meantime, heat a large non-stick pan over medium-high heat with the olive oil.
4. Add the zucchini.
5. Cook until the zucchini is golden and tender, about 10 minutes.
6. In a large mixing bowl, combine the millet, parsley, chives, lemon zest, and lemon juice, and set it aside.
7. Add the chickpeas to a food processor and pulse until ground.
8. Transfer ground chickpeas to the mixing bowl.
9. Now add the zucchini, salt, cumin, egg whites, and rice flour.
10. Mix together with your hands until well combined.
11. Divide the mixture into 4 patties.
12. Lightly coat the bottom of the skillet with the coconut oil.
13. Add the veggie fritters and cook them until a golden crust forms, about 5 to 6 minutes.
14. Flip them to the other side and cook them another 5 minutes, or until that side is also golden.

Per serving: Calories: 429 Protein: 11g Carbs: 46g Fiber: 6g Sugar: 4g Fat: 23g

Grilled Citrus Fennel Hearts

SERVES 2 / PREP TIME: 10 MINUTES / COOK TIME: 20 MINUTES

These scrumptious fennel hearts pair well with a crunchy green salad.

---

2 small fennel hearts, sliced
2 tablespoons extra virgin olive oil
2 tablespoons fresh lemon juice
1/2 lemon, zest only
A pinch of salt to taste

---

1. Place the fennel hearts, oil, lemon juice, and zest in a shallow dish,
2. Season everything with salt.
3. Toss to coat well.
4. Let the dish stand to marinate for at least 10 minutes.
5. To cook, toss the fennel slices on a barbecue grill or a non stick pan for 5-10 minutes on each side, turning several times with tongs, until they are crisp-tender and the edges are slightly charred.
6. Drizzle the hearts with additional olive oil to serve.

Per serving: Calories: 196 Protein: 3g Carbs: 18g Sugar: 9g Fat: 15g

Tossed Brown Rice and Spinach Bowl

SERVES 2 / PREP TIME: 10 MINUTES / COOK TIME: 35 MINUTES

This filling and tasty rice bowl is sure to perk up your afternoon!

---

1 cup brown rice
2 cups boiling water
A pinch of salt
2 medium carrots, peeled and sliced

4 tbsp lemon juice
1 tbsp olive oil
2 cups fresh spinach
1 tbsp olive oil
1 tbsp apple cider vinegar
A pinch of salt
1 handful pumpkin seeds

---

1. Place the rice in a pot with the boiling water and a pinch of salt.
2. Simmer on low heat for 20 minutes until all the water has been absorbed.
3. Meanwhile, steam the carrots over the saucepan with the rice in for 20 minutes.
4. Place the carrots in a large salad bowl.
5. Stir in the lemon juice.
6. Next, it's time to heat 1 tbsp olive oil in a pan over medium-high heat.
7. Add the spinach and sauté for 5 minutes, or until the spinach has wilted.
8. Remove the spinach.
9. Mix 1 tbsp olive oil, vinegar, and salt together in a small bowl to make the dressing.
10. Add all the ingredients together into the salad bowl with the carrots.
11. Toss to coat and serve.

Per serving: Calories: 523 Protein: 10 Carbs: 80 Fiber: 8 Sugar: 5 Fat: 19
(Unsaturated: 16 Saturated: 3)

Quinoa and Eggplant Boats

SERVES 4 / PREP TIME: 5 MINUTES / COOK TIME: 55 MINUTES

Stuffed and roasted eggplants.

---

2 medium eggplants, halved lengthwise
2 tbsp olive oil
2 tsp kosher salt
2 cups fresh spinach, washed
5 oz crumbled goat cheese
1 cup quinoa, cooked
3 tbsp gluten-free breadcrumbs

1 lemon, zest only
1 tbsp chopped fresh parsley
A pinch of salt to taste

---

1. Preheat the oven to 400 degrees.
2. Fill a large pan of water and bring to the boil over high heat.
3. Add the eggplant halves and cook for 4-5 minutes.
4. Drain the eggplant well.
5. Pat dry with paper towels.
6. Place the eggplant on a baking sheet.
7. Brush the eggplant with half the olive oil.
8. Bake in the oven for 20-25 minutes, or until tender and golden.
9. Remove the eggplant from the oven.
10. Scoop out the flesh, leaving about 1/4 inch of flesh attached to the skin.
11. Set the skins aside.
12. Now roughly chop the eggplant flesh that you scooped out.
13. Meanwhile, heat the remaining oil in a large frying pan.
14. Add the eggplant flesh to the pan and sauté for a few minutes.
15. Add the spinach and cook for 3-4 minutes, or until the spinach is wilted, stirring frequently.
16. Remove the pan from the heat.
17. Stir in the cheese and cooked quinoa.
18. In a separate bowl, mix together the breadcrumbs, lemon zest, parsley, and salt.
19. Spoon the spinach mixture into the eggplant halves.
20. Sprinkle the top of each eggplant with the breadcrumb mixture.
21. Return this to the oven.
22. Bake for 10-15 minutes, or until the topping is golden.

Per serving: Calories: 325 Protein: 14g Carbs: 28g Fiber: 10g Sugar: 11g Fat: 19g

Carrot Infused Potato Gnocchi

SERVES 4 / PREP TIME: 20 MINUTES / COOK TIME: 30 MINUTES

This simple carrot and potato gnocchi is sure to delight everyone's taste buds!

1 oz fresh cilantro, torn
1 tbsp garlic infused oil
1 tbsp extra-virgin olive oil
7 oz potatoes
2 cups carrots, peeled and sliced
2 egg whites
1 1/4 cup brown rice flour
2 tbsp crumbled feta cheese

1. For the sauce, add the cilantro to a food processor with the two oils.
2. Blend the cilantro mixture to a paste.
3. Set aside for later.
4. Peel and boil the potatoes in double the amount of water for 20 minutes, or until soft.
5. Add the carrots to the pan after 5 minutes then drain.
6. Add the cooked carrot and potato to a mixing bowl.
7. Mash the cooked potato and carrots with a masher or a large fork until the mixture is smooth.
8. Add the egg whites, rice flour, and feta cheese to the carrots and potatoes.
9. Mix everything together with your hands until you have a smooth dough.
10. Divide the dough into four balls.
11. On a lightly floured surface or table, roll each ball of potato dough into a long sausage shape about 1 inch thick.
12. Then, using a table knife, cut each roll into 1 inch pieces to form gnocchi.
13. Press each gnocchi with a fork to make a ridged pattern.
14. Fill a large pan with water and bring to a boil with a pinch of salt.
15. Place 10 gnocchi at a time carefully into the water.
16. Boil for 30 seconds.
17. The gnocchi will rise to the surface of the water when they are cooked.
18. Remove the gnocchi from the water with a slotted spoon.
19. Place the cooked gnocchi into warm bowls.
20. Stir in a teaspoonful of the sauce to serve.

Hint: If the dough becomes sticky, you can simply add more flour.

Per serving: Calories: 314 Protein: 7g Carbs: 51g Fiber: 5g Sugar: 4g Fat: 9g

Vegetarian Feta and Tomato Quiche

SERVES 4 / PREP TIME: 1 HOUR / COOK TIME: 1 HOUR

This very traditional recipe is well worth the extra effort to bake from scratch!

3 oz rice flour	2 tbsp cold water
3 oz fine cornmeal	1 cup tomatoes, diced
3 oz potato flour	1 tbsp olive oil
1 tsp xanthan gum	A pinch of salt to taste
A pinch of salt	½ cup feta cheese
5 oz coconut oil, cold	3 egg whites
1 egg white, lightly beaten	1 tbsp basil leaves, torn

1. Sift the rice flour, fine cornmeal, potato flour, xanthan gum, and salt into a bowl and mix well.
2. Cut the cold oil into cubes and gently work into the flour mixture with your finger tips until mixed in.
3. Make a well in the center of the flour; add 1 egg white and 1 tbsp water.
4. Mix the pastry dough together using a fork and roll into a ball with your hands.
5. On a lightly floured board, gently knead the dough with the heel of your hand for a few minutes to form a silky-smooth ball. Flatten the ball slightly before wrapping it in plastic wrap and refrigerating for about 30 minutes.
6. Roll out the pastry dough into a large circular shape and lift up with a rolling pin. Drape over the pie pan so that the crust hangs over the sides a little.
7. Gently push the pastry into the corners of the pie pan. Chill the pie pan in the fridge or freezer for a further 20 minutes.
8. Meanwhile, preheat oven to 400 degrees.
9. Add the tomatoes, the olive oil, and the salt to a baking sheet and place in the oven.
10. Remove the pie crust from the fridge and lightly prick the bottom of the crust all over with a fork.
11. Cover the dough with a circle of aluminum foil or parchment paper and fill it with ceramic baking beans - blind bake for 20 minutes.
12. Remove the crust from the oven and take out the foil and beans before returning to oven for 5-10 minutes, or until light brown. Remove crust and tomatoes from oven.
13. In the meantime, beat 3 egg whites in a large bowl and stir in most of the basil.
14. Sprinkle half the cheese over the bottom, then layer the tomatoes, pour over the egg whites, and sprinkle the rest of the cheese over the top.
15. Bake for 20-25 minutes, or until set and golden brown - serve!

Per serving: Calories: 535 Protein: 11g Carbs: 54g Sugar: 3g Fat: 32g

Zesty Lime Eggplant

SERVES 4 / PREP TIME: 10 MINUTES / COOK TIME: 25 MINUTES

This sweet and zesty quinoa is filling and satisfying!

---

2 tbsp coconut oil
2 tbsp pure maple syrup
2 small eggplants, cut into wedges
1 red bell pepper, de-seeded and diced
1 ½ cups red quinoa
1 lime, zest and juice
1 tbsp fresh mint leaves, chopped

---

1. Add the quinoa to a pan with 3 cups boiling water.
2. Simmer on medium heat for 20 minutes.
3. Mix together the oil and maple syrup.
4. Next, drizzle half the syrup mixture over the eggplants and pepper.
5. Heat a non stick frying pan over medium heat.
6. Cook the vegetables for 10-15 minutes, turning them until they are lightly charred and cooked through.
7. Drain the quinoa.
8. Next, pour the remaining syrup mixture, the lime juice, the lime zest, and the mint leaves over the quinoa and toss to coat.
9. Serve the quinoa with the roasted vegetables on top.

Per serving: Calories: 395 Protein: 11g Carbs: 66g Fiber: 14g Sugar: 20g Fat: 11g

Parsley and Quinoa Tabbouleh

SERVES 2 / PREP TIME: 5 MINUTES / COOK TIME: 20 MINUTES

This healthy tabbouleh recipe will add flavor to any Mediterranean dish!

---

1 cup quinoa
2 cups water
1 lemon, juice and zest
2 tbsp olive oil
2 tbsp fresh mint, chopped
2 tbsp fresh flat-leaf parsley, chopped

1 tbsp green onions (green tips only), chopped
½ cucumber, diced
A pinch of salt to taste
1/4 cup shredded lettuce

---

1. Rinse the quinoa well under cold water.
2. Place into a pan with 2 cups boiling water over high heat.
3. Bring the pan to a boil.
4. Cover the quinoa, reduce the heat, and gently simmer for 20 minutes, or until most of the water has been soaked up.
5. Turn off the heat and leave the lid on so it can steam for a few minutes.
6. Drain any remaining water.
7. Into the quinoa, stir the lemon juice and the olive oil.
8. Allow to cool fully.
9. Finally, stir in the other ingredients before serving.

Per serving: Calories: 440 Protein: 12g Carbs: 58g Fiber: 8g Sugar: 4g Fat: 19g

Mediterranean Grilled Vegetables

SERVES 5 / PREP TIME: 5 MINUTES / COOK TIME: 30 MINUTES

So simple yet so scrumptious!

---

2 large eggplants, cubed
2 red bell peppers, seeded and sliced
into 4 pieces
4 small zucchinis
4 large tomatoes

4 tbsp olive oil
1 tbsp red wine vinegar
1 tsp coconut sugar
1/8 cup fresh basil, torn
1 tbsp garlic infused oil
1 tbsp chopped chives (green tips only)
A pinch of salt to taste

---

1. Preheat the broiler/grill to medium-low heat.
2. Spread all of the vegetables out across a lined baking sheet.
3. In a bowl, stir together the rest of the ingredients.
4. Pour this over the vegetables and stir to coat.
5. Broil/grill for 25-30 minutes until soft and lightly browned.
6. Remove and enjoy hot or allow to cool and refrigerate to serve as an antipasti on a hot summer's day!

Per serving: Calories: 237 Protein: 5g Carbs: 25 Fiber: 10g Sugar: 17g Fat: 15g

Italian Eggplant Lasagna

SERVES 6 / PREP TIME: 10 MINUTES / COOK TIME: 1 HOUR

This delectable lasagna is delicious with the thick bubbling tomato sauce.

---

2 tbsp olive oil, plus extra for brushing
2 fresh thyme sprigs
8 large fresh sage leaves, finely chopped
4 cans diced tomatoes
3 tbsp red wine vinegar
3 tbsp coconut sugar

1 large eggplant, sliced lengthways as thinly as you can
1 cup crumbled goat cheese
1 tbsp dried oregano
1 tbsp dried basil
A pinch of salt to taste

---

1. Preheat the oven to 400 degrees.
2. Heat the oil in a large skillet.
3. Add the thyme and sage, cooking gently for a few minutes.
4. Add in the diced tomatoes, vinegar, and sugar.
5. Gently simmer the tomatoes for 20-25 minutes, or until slightly thickened, and remove from the heat.
6. Meanwhile, heat a skillet over medium heat.
7. While it's heating up, brush the eggplant slices on both sides with the extra olive oil.
8. Add to the skillet for 4-5 minutes, or until lightly charred on both sides.
9. Into an oven dish, spread a little of the tomato sauce over the bottom.
10. Top the sauce with a layer of eggplant slices.
11. Spoon over this a bit more sauce.
12. Next sprinkle over the sauce a little of the goat cheese, oregano, basil, and salt.
13. Repeat this process until you have several layers of eggplant and sauce.
14. Finish the top layer with the last of the tomato sauce.
15. Bake the lasagna for 30-40 minutes, or until the top is crisp and golden.
16. Leave to cool for 10 minutes before serving.

Per serving: Calories: 251 Protein: 9g Carbs: 20g Fiber: 8g Sugar: 14g Fat: 17g

Spanish Potato Omelet

SERVES 2 / PREP TIME: 5 MINUTES / COOK TIME: 40 MINUTES

A slow cooked chunky omelet, typical of a Spanish tapas dish.

---

10 egg whites
A pinch of salt to taste
1 tbsp olive oil
2 zucchinis, finely chopped
4 roasted red peppers, drained and finely chopped
1 tbsp garlic infused oil
1 white potato, peeled, boiled and sliced

1 cup fresh spinach, washed
1 tbsp dried oregano
4 tbsp chives (green tips only), chopped
1 tbsp olive oil

---

1. Whisk the egg whites lightly in a bowl.
2. Season with the salt.
3. Now heat the oil in a large frying pan.
4. Add the zucchinis.
5. Sauté gently for about 10 minutes, or until softened.
6. Let the zucchini cool a little.
7. Add to the egg whites.
8. Now add the roasted peppers to the egg whites, along with the garlic oil.
9. Into the hot pan, cook the potato slices for 5-10 minutes.
10. Pour the egg mixture into the pan and cover with a lid.
11. Turn down the burner to the lowest heat setting.
12. Leave to cook without disturbing for 15-20 minutes.
13. Occasionally check to ensure it's not burning, by gently lifting the edge with a spatula.
14. It will be cooked when the top of the omelet is no longer runny and you can easily lift it out of the pan with your spatula.
15. Serve the omelet with the spinach, oregano, and chives dressed in the remaining olive oil.

Hint: You can double check that the omelet is cooked through by poking a knife into the center - it should pull out clean.

Per serving: Calories: 475 Protein: 26g Carbs: 48g Fiber: 9g Sugar: 21g Fat: 22g

Cheesy Zucchini and Lemon Risotto

SERVES 4 / PREP TIME: 10 MINUTES / COOK TIME: 35 MINUTES

A superb risotto that tastes fresh and zesty.

---

4 zucchinis
Olive oil cooking spray
½ cup risotto rice
1 lemon, zest and juice
4 cups hot low sodium vegetable stock
¼ cup feta cheese, crumbled
2 tbsp cashew milk

---

1. Grate 2 of the zucchinis with a cheese grater into a bowl or on a plate.
2. Dice the other 2 zucchinis.
3. Spray a skillet with olive oil spray over medium heat.
4. Add the grated zucchini and the rice to the skillet.
5. Turn up the heat to medium-high and stir for 1-2 minutes.
6. Add the lemon juice and a ladle of the hot stock.
7. Bring this to a boil over medium-high heat while stirring constantly.
8. When the liquid has just about been absorbed, add another ladle of stock.
9. Continue until all of the stock is in the skillet.
10. Cook for 20-25 minutes, or until the rice is just tender and creamy.
11. Stir in the feta cheese and cashew milk.
12. Cover the skillet with a lid or baking sheet.
13. Set aside for 5 minutes while you cook the remaining zucchini.
14. Spray a small frying pan with olive oil spray.
15. Add the diced zucchini.
16. Sauté over high heat for 2-3 minutes, or until golden and just softened.
17. Divide the risotto among 4 shallow bowls or plates.
18. Sprinkle the diced zucchini and lemon zest over the bowls to serve.

Per serving: Calories: 129 Protein: 5g Carbs: 21g Sugar: 9g Fat: 3g

Zucchini Shepherd's Pie

SERVES 2 / PREP TIME: 10 MINUTES / COOK TIME: 1 HOUR

You don't miss the meat in this delicious zucchini version of traditional shepherd's pie!

1 tbsp olive oil
2 zucchinis, diced
2 carrots, diced
1 stalk celery, chopped
2 bay leaves
1 tbsp dried thyme
1 tbsp chopped chives (green tips only)
2 cups low FODMAP vegetable stock
2 tbsp tomato paste

2 cups white potatoes, peeled and diced
1 cup rice milk
A pinch of salt and pepper to taste

1. Preheat the oven to 375 degrees.
2. To make the sauce, heat the olive oil in a pan over medium heat.
3. In the warm oil, sauté all the vegetables for 10 minutes, or until soft and golden.
4. Stir in the herbs and chives.
5. Now pour the stock over the vegetables.
6. Simmer for 20 minutes over medium-low heat, or until the vegetables are very soft.
7. Meanwhile, place the potatoes into a pan of water.
8. Boil them for about 15 minutes, or until tender.
9. Now take the pan of vegetables off the heat and stir in the tomato paste.
10. Drain the potatoes, return to the pot, and mash with the milk and the salt.
11. Pour the vegetable mixture into a deep baking dish.
12. Top with the mashed potatoes.
13. Use a fork to score the top of the potato mixture, creating ridges.
14. Bake the casserole for 30 minutes, or until the top is golden brown.
15. Season with salt and pepper to taste and serve.

Hint: You can add in other low FODMAP veggies to your taste.

Per serving: Calories: 328 Protein: 12g Carbs: 51g Fiber: 9g Sugar: 17g Fat: 10g

STOCKS, SOUPS AND STEWS

Classic Low FODMAP Chicken Stock

SERVES 6 / PREP TIME: 30 MINUTES / COOK TIME: 2 HOURS

This scrumptious chicken stock is great to have on hand year round!

2-3 lb whole chicken, cut apart at the thighs, breasts and legs
2 celery stalks with leaves, diced
2 medium carrots, chopped
2 bay leaves

½ tsp dried parsley
½ tsp dried oregano
¼ tsp dried basil
1 dash pink Himalayan sea salt
8 cups cold water

---

1. Place all the ingredients into a heavy pot.
2. Bring the stock to a boil over high heat.
3. Reduce the heat and skim any foam off the top with a knife.
4. Cover the stock and simmer for 2 hours.
5. Next, gently remove the chicken from the stock.
6. Set it aside on a chopping board.
7. Strain the rest of the stock into a glass jar or bowl through a fine meshed sieve or muslin cloth.
8. Discard the vegetables.
9. Refrigerate the stock for 8 hours or overnight.
10. Once cooled, you can skim the fat from the surface.

Hint: Keep this stock in an airtight container in the fridge for 2-3 days or the freezer for 2-3 weeks to use in future recipes. Portion up first to make individual servings easier.

Hint: Carve up the chicken meat and serve cold with salads or sandwiches, or flake with a knife and fork and add back into a portion of the chicken stock to make a delicious hot chunky chicken soup.

Per serving: Calories: 128 Protein: 8g Carbs: 14g Sugar: 6g Fat: 4g

Low FODMAP Vegetable Stock

SERVES 6 / PREP TIME: 30 MINUTES / COOK TIME: 2 HOURS

This refreshing stock is perfect as a rainy day soup or as an addition to many of the recipes in this cookbook.

2 stalks celery, roughly chopped
6 large carrots, roughly chopped
2 turnips, roughly chopped
3 bay leaves
1 bunch fresh parsley, washed and roughly chopped
2 sprigs fresh rosemary
2 sprigs fresh thyme
1 sprig fresh oregano

1 bunch fresh green onions, chopped (green tips only)
5 whole white peppercorns
A pinch of salt
4 liters cold water

1. In a large soup pot, bring all the ingredients to a boil over high heat.
2. Reduce the heat to a simmer and cook, uncovered, for 2 hours.
3. Occasionally skim the surface to remove any foam that rises.
4. Next, pour the stock through a wire mesh strainer into a glass jar.
5. Discard the vegetables and herbs.
6. Allow the stock to cool, seal, and refrigerate.

Hint: Keep this stock in an airtight container in the fridge for 2-3 days or the freezer for 2-3 weeks to use in future recipes. Portion up first to make individual servings easier.

Per serving: Calories: 41 Protein: 1g Carbs: 9g Fiber: 3g Sugar: 4g Fat: 0g

Low FODMAP Seafood Stock

SERVES 8 / PREP TIME: 10 MINUTES / COOK TIME: 1 HOUR

This simple stock is good to have around to make recipes interesting!

---

3 lb fish bones, including heads
6 cups water
1 large carrot, chopped
3 celery stalks, including the leafy top,
sliced
A pinch of salt

---

1. Place the fish bones in the water and bring it to a boil over high heat.
2. Simmer the bones for 20 minutes.
3. Now pour the water through a wire mesh strainer into a container or serving jar
4. Return the water to the pan and add the vegetables and seasoning.
5. Bring it to a boil over high heat.
6. Turn down the heat and simmer the stock for 45 minutes.
7. Strain it one last time into jars.
8. Once it has cooled down, you can store it in the fridge or freezer in small quantities.

Hint: Keep this stock in an airtight container in the fridge for 2-3 days or the freezer for 2-3 weeks to use in future recipes. Portion up first to make individual servings easier.

Per serving: Calories: 39 Protein: 4g Carbs: 2g Sugar: 1g Fat: 1g

Sweet Collard Green Stew

SERVES 4 / PREP TIME: 5 MINUTES / COOK TIME: 50 MINUTES

Packed with vitamins!

---

1 tbsp olive oil
1 tsp smoked paprika
1 tsp cumin
6 medium carrots, sliced
1/4 cup water
6 cups dandelion or collard greens, loosely packed
3 cups water
1 (15 oz) can diced tomatoes, no salt

added
1 (6 oz) can tomato paste, no salt added
3 tbsp low sodium soy sauce or tamari
3 tbsp fresh lemon juice
1 tbsp pure maple syrup
1 tsp salt
1/2 tsp dried oregano

---

1. Add the oil to a large cooking pot.
2. Add the paprika and cumin.
3. Turn the heat on to medium.
4. Add the carrots and 1/4 cup water.
5. Place the lid on the pot and cook for 10 minutes, stirring occasionally.
6. Stem the greens whilst the carrots cook.
7. Stir in the rest of the ingredients.
8. Raise the heat to medium-high.
9. Now cover the pot and bring the stew to a boil.
10. Turn the heat down to medium.
11. Uncover the stew and leave to simmer for 30-35 minutes.
12. Ladle the stew into bowls to serve.

Per serving: Calories: 324 Protein: 12g Carbs: 58g Fiber: 13g Sugar: 16 Fat: 6g

Creamy Carrot and Potato Bisque

SERVES 4 / PREP TIME: 5 MINUTES / COOK TIME: 30 MINUTES

This bisque is made creamy by the softened potatoes and carrots.

---

2 medium potatoes
2 large carrots
1 1/2 tbsp fresh cilantro, loosely chopped
1 tbsp garlic infused oil
1 tbsp olive oil
1/2 cup green onions (green tips only), sliced

3 cups low FODMAP chicken stock/ vegetable stock
1 tbsp olive oil
1 tbsp dried oregano
1/2 cup unsweetened light coconut milk
A pinch of salt to taste

---

1. Peel and cut the potatoes and carrots into small pieces.
2. Roughly chop the fresh cilantro.
3. Reserve a few pinches for the garnish later.
4. Place the garlic infused oil and olive oil in a large saucepan.
5. Over low heat, cook the green onions for 1 to 2 minutes, stirring occasionally.
6. Next, add the potatoes and carrots to the saucepan.
7. Cook the vegetables over low heat for 5 minutes, stirring occasionally.
8. Add the stock to the saucepan.
9. Turn up the heat to medium-high and bring the soup to a rolling boil.
10. Put the lid on the saucepan and allow the soup to simmer for 10 to 15 minutes, or until the vegetables are tender.
11. Meanwhile, heat the olive oil in a skillet.
12. Add the fresh cilantro and cook for one minute, then remove it from the heat.
13. Add this to the soup.
14. Once the vegetables are tender, remove the soup from the heat and let it cool for 10 minutes.
15. Transfer the soup to a food processor or blender, in batches if needed, and process the soup until smooth.
16. Rinse out the soup pot and then return the soup to it.
17. Over low heat, mix in the milk and season it with a pinch of salt to taste.
18. Serve the soup warm with a sprinkle of fresh cilantro.

Per serving: Calories: 193 Protein: 6g Carbs: 18g Sugar: 2g Fat: 13g

Roasted Pepper and Parsnip Soup

SERVES 4 / PREP TIME: 10 MINUTES / COOK TIME: 35 MINUTES

The sweetness of the peppers and parsnips is released during the roasting process of this delectable soup recipe.

2 medium parsnips, peeled and chopped
2 large carrots, peeled and chopped
2 red bell peppers, seeded and cut into strips
1 tbsp coconut oil
A pinch of salt and pepper to taste
4 cups low FODMAP vegetable stock
1 (15 oz) can diced tomatoes

1 tbsp garlic-infused olive oil
1 tbsp paprika
3 tbsp fresh parsley, torn

1. Preheat the oven to 400 degrees.
2. Place the parsnips, carrots, and red peppers on a baking sheet.
3. Drizzle over the oil and season the vegetables with salt and pepper.
4. Toss this mixture so that the veggies are well coated with oil.
5. Place the sheet in the oven and roast it for 20 to 25 minutes, or until golden and soft.
6. Toss the mixture once while cooking.
7. Once the veggies are roasted, transfer them to a blender.
8. Add half of the stock and the tomatoes to the blender.
9. Blend everything together until smooth.
10. Transfer the soup back into the large saucepan.
11. Place the saucepan over medium heat.
12. Stir into the soup the other half of the stock, the garlic infused oil, and the paprika.
13. Season to taste if required.
14. Allow the soup to heat through for 10 minutes.
15. Serve the soup with parsley sprinkled on top.

Per serving: Calories: 188 Protein: 5g Carbs: 27g Fiber: 8g Sugar: 12g Fat: 8g

Slow Cooker Chicken Soup

SERVES 4 / PREP TIME: 10 MINUTES / COOK TIME: 6-7 HOURS SLOW COOKER

This classic dish tastes wonderful after cooking all day—and smells good too!

Olive oil cooking spray
1 lb skinless chicken breasts
2 large carrots, peeled and chopped
2 parsnips, peeled and chopped
1/2 cup chives (green tips only), finely chopped
2 tbsp garlic infused oil
1 tbsp fresh lemon juice
1/2 tsp dried thyme
1/2 tsp dried rosemary

1/2 tsp dried oregano
2 dried bay leaves
4 cups low FODMAP chicken stock
A pinch of salt to taste
3 tbsp fresh parsley, finely chopped
1 tbsp fresh cilantro, chopped

1. Spray the slow cooker dish with cooking spray.
2. Line the bottom of the slow cooker with the chicken breasts. Cover them with the carrots, parsnips, chives, garlic infused oil, fresh lemon juice, thyme, rosemary, oregano, and bay leaves.
3. Cover everything with the low FODMAP chicken stock.
4. Season with a pinch of salt to taste.
5. Place the lid on the slow cooker.
6. Cook on Low for 6 to 7 hours.
7. Just before serving, shred the chicken breasts using two forks.
8. Dish the hot chicken soup into bowls and sprinkle with the parsley and cilantro.

Per serving: Calories: 276 Protein: 32g Carbs: 20g Fiber: 4g Sugar: 6g Fat: 8g

Quick Oriental Chicken Soup

SERVES 4 / PREP TIME: 5 MINUTES / COOK TIME: 35 MINUTES

This tasty Oriental-inspired chicken soup will comfort you on sick days and any other for that matter!

---

1 tbsp olive oil
2 (5 oz) chicken breasts, sliced
A pinch of salt to taste
2 cups low FODMAP chicken stock
1 tsp powdered ginger
½ tsp turmeric
1 tbsp sliced chives (green ends only), sliced
½ cup fresh spinach leaves
1 tbsp low sodium soy sauce

1 tsp fish sauce
5 large tomatoes, halved
7 oz rice noodles, cooked

---

1. Heat the oil in a large pot over medium-high heat.
2. Add the chicken breast slices and season them with the salt.
3. Sauté for 15-20 minutes, or until golden-brown and cooked through.
4. In a separate pan, bring the stock to a boil.
5. To the stock, add the ginger, turmeric, chives, spinach, soy sauce, fish sauce, and tomatoes.
6. Reduce the heat and allow to simmer for 4-5 minutes, or until heated through.
7. Now add to the stock, the cooked chicken and rice noodles.
8. Continue to heat for 10 minutes until the mixture is warmed through.
9. Ladle into bowls to serve.

Hint: Check that the juices of the chicken run clear when pierced in the thickest part of the center.

Per serving: Calories: 323 Protein: 21g Carbs: 44g Fiber: 4g Sugar: 5g Fat: 7g

Cream of Tomato Soup

SERVES 2 / PREP TIME: 5 MINUTES / COOK TIME: 30 MINUTES

Potatoes are the secret to this creamy yet healthy tomato soup.

3 tbsp olive oil
2 celery stalks, chopped
2 small carrots, peeled and chopped
1 large white potato, peeled and diced
4 bay leaves

5 tbsp tomato paste
1 tsp dried oregano
2 tbsp coconut sugar
3 tbsp red wine vinegar
4 cups tomatoes, diced
1 cup low FODMAP chicken stock

1. Add the oil, celery, carrots, potato, and bay leaves to a large pot over medium heat.
2. Stir in the tomato paste, oregano, sugar, vinegar, tomatoes, and stock.
3. Cover the soup and simmer for 25 minutes, or until the potato is tender.
4. Remove the bay leaves and allow to cool slightly.
5. Next, purée the soup with a stick blender until it is very smooth.
6. Ladle into 2 bowls to serve.

Hint: If you don't have a stick blender, ladle the soup into a blender in batches.

Per serving: Calories: 495 Protein: 12g Carbs: 68g Fiber: 13g Sugar: 24g Fat: 22g

Puréed Moroccan Zucchini Soup

SERVES 2 / PREP TIME: 5 MINUTES / COOK TIME: 40 MINUTES

This creamy soup is marked by the North African flavors of cinnamon and turmeric.

1 tbsp olive oil
2 stalks celery, chopped
2 zucchinis, sliced
2 cups tomatoes, diced
2 tbsp coconut flour
½ tsp turmeric
½ tsp ground cumin

2 cups low FODMAP vegetable stock

1. Heat the olive oil in a large pan over medium heat.
2. Add the celery and zucchini.
3. Sauté for 5 minutes over medium heat, stirring occasionally.
4. Add the tomatoes and coconut flour.
5. Cook for 2 minutes while stirring.
6. Add the turmeric, cumin, and stock.
7. Cover and simmer the soup for 30 minutes.
8. Allow to cool slightly.
9. Purée the soup with a stick blender until very smooth.
10. Ladle into 2 bowls to serve.

Hint: If you don't have a stick blender, ladle the soup into a blender in batches.

Per serving: Calories: 155 Protein: 3g Carbs: 16g Sugar: 5g Fat: 8g

Creamy Carrot and Potato Soup

SERVES 2 / PREP TIME: 10 MINUTES / COOK TIME: 1 HOUR

This delightful creamy soup is sure to be a crowd pleaser!

---

3 tbsp olive oil
2 celery stalks, chopped
2 carrots, sliced
1 white potato, peeled and diced
1 dried bay leaf
1/2 tsp dried oregano

2 cups tomatoes, diced
1 tbsp coconut sugar
1 tbsp red wine vinegar
2 cups low FODMAP vegetable stock
½ cup cashew milk

---

1. Add the oil and celery to a large pot over medium heat.
2. Sauté the celery gently until it has softened, about 5 minutes.
3. Add the carrots and diced potato.
4. Cook for 3 more minutes.
5. Now add all the remaining ingredients except the milk.
6. Bring the soup to a simmer.
7. Cover the soup and simmer for 30 minutes.
8. After this, allow it to simmer uncovered for 20 minutes.
9. Remove the bay leaves.
10. Allow to cool slightly.
11. Use a stick blender or regular blender to purée the soup into a creamy consistency.
12. Add the cashew milk and stir well.
13. Ladle into 2 bowls to serve.

Per serving: Calories: 353 Protein: 4 Carbs: 38 Sugar: 17 Fat: 22

Roasted Bell Pepper Bisque

SERVES 4 / PREP TIME: 10 MINUTES / COOK TIME: 45 MINUTES

The rich flavors of bell peppers and eggplant shine through in this creamy bisque.

---

2 large tomatoes, halved
1 red bell pepper, roughly chopped
1 yellow bell pepper, roughly chopped
2 celery stalks, diced
1 eggplant, roughly chopped
2 tbsp coconut oil
1 tbsp balsamic vinegar
2 tbsp coconut sugar
1 tsp dried thyme

1 tbsp dried oregano
1 tsp dried basil
2 cups low FODMAP vegetable Stock
A pinch of salt to taste

---

1. Preheat the oven to 400 degrees.
2. Peel and roughly chop the vegetables.
3. Place them together into a roasting pan.
4. In a separate bowl, mix together the coconut oil, vinegar, sugar, thyme, oregano, and basil.
5. Hint: you may need to warm the coconut oil if it's solid - the palms of your hands should be sufficient!
6. Drizzle this mixture over the vegetables.
7. Cover and transfer the roasting pan to the oven.
8. Roast the vegetables for 35 minutes, or until they are tender and golden brown.
9. Heat the vegetable stock in your stockpot.
10. Add the roasted vegetables to the soup.
11. Once it is boiling, reduce the heat and simmer for 10 minutes.
12. Turn off the heat and let the soup cool down for a few minutes.
13. Purée the ingredients with a hand blender in the stockpot, or in batches in a food processor.
14. Return the soup to the pan.
15. Season to taste with salt.
16. Ladle into 4 bowls to serve.

Per serving: Calories: 151 Protein: 4g Carbs: 20g Fiber: 7g Sugar: 12g Fat: 8g

Pumpkin Sage Bisque

SERVES 4 / PREP TIME: 15 MINUTES / COOK TIME: 1 HOUR

The delicious blend of pumpkin and sage makes a perfect autumn dinner!

1 (5 lb) pumpkin, gutted (use canned
alternatively
1 tbsp coconut oil
½ tsp cumin
½ tsp turmeric
A pinch of salt to taste
6 cups low FODMAP vegetable stock
8 fresh sage Leaves

1. Using a sharp knife and a spoon, carefully hollow out the pumpkin, removing the flesh and setting it aside on a chopping board.
2. Roughly chop the scooped-out pumpkin flesh.
3. Heat a pan over low heat and add the oil.
4. Add the pumpkin flesh, cumin, turmeric, and salt.
5. Increase the heat to high.
6. Add the stock and sage leaves and bring to a rolling boil.
7. Lower the heat to medium and cover the pan with the lid.
8. Cook for 40-45 minutes, stirring occasionally to prevent it from burning, until the pumpkin is cooked through.
9. Remove the soup from the heat and allow to cool slightly.
10. Use a stick blender, or transfer the soup to a food processor in batches, and blend until smooth.
11. Return the soup to the pan.
12. Ladle it into bowls to serve.

Per serving: Calories: 104 Protein: 5g Carbs: 15g Fiber: 3g Sugar: 4g Fat: 4g

Fresh Parsley and Potato Turkey Stew

SERVES 2 / PREP TIME: 10 MINUTES / COOK TIME: 1 HOUR

This unique stew is perfect for any winter evening meal!

1 tbsp olive oil
2 (6 oz) turkey breasts
A pinch of salt and pepper to taste
2 stalks celery, diced
2 carrots, diced
1 tsp dried oregano

1 tsp dried cilantro
2 cups low FODMAP chicken stock
2 medium white potatoes, peeled and cubed
1 bunch fresh parsley, roughly chopped

1. Heat a stock pot over high heat.
2. Add the oil.
3. While the oil is heating, season the turkey with the salt and pepper.
4. Add the turkey breasts to the pan and brown each side for 7-8 minutes.
5. Turn the heat down to medium and add the celery, carrots, oregano, and cilantro.
6. Pour in the stock, mixing well.
7. Add the potatoes and stir.
8. Reduce the heat, cover, and simmer for 1 hour, stirring occasionally.
9. Remove the turkey from the stew and leave to one side to cool slightly.
10. Meanwhile, shred the meat after it has cooled down.
11. Add the meat back to the pan and stir well.
12. Once you are ready to serve the stew, stir in the chopped parsley.
13. Serve hot.

Hint: Use dinner forks or meat claws to shred the turkey meat.

Per serving: Calories: 429 Protein: 44g Carbs: 42g Fiber: 6g Sugar: 3g Fat: 9g

Gluten Free Paprika Chicken Goulash

SERVES 4 / PREP TIME: 10 MINUTES / COOK TIME: 35 MINUTES

This healthy goulash is served over rice noodles for a delicious dinner!

2 tbsp olive oil
2 carrots, diced
2 stalks celery, diced
2 medium white potatoes, peeled and diced
4 (5 oz) skinless chicken breasts, diced
1 tbsp smoked paprika
1 tbsp golden flax meal

4 cups low FODMAP chicken stock
1 tbsp tomato paste
A pinch of salt to taste
4 large tomatoes, diced
1 red bell pepper, seeded and diced
2 tbsp green onion (tips only), sliced
1 (8 oz) package rice noodles, cooked

1. Heat half the oil in a large frying pan over medium heat.
2. Gently sauté the carrots and celery for 5 minutes, or until softened.
3. Add the potatoes and sauté for 2 more minutes.
4. Remove the vegetables from the pan and set them to one side.
5. Add the remaining oil to the pan and sear the diced chicken on all sides
6. Return the vegetables to the pan and sprinkle in the paprika and flax meal.
7. Cook this for 5-7 minutes, stirring frequently until chicken is golden.
8. Gradually stir in the stock, tomato paste, and salt.
9. Turn the heat to high, bring to a boil, stirring occasionally, then lower the heat.
10. Add the diced tomatoes to the soup and simmer for 20 minutes.
11. In a separate saucepan, blanch the bell pepper in boiling water for 4 minutes.
12. Drain it and add the pepper to the soup.
13. Cook it for 5-10 minutes, or until the chicken is tender.
14. Pour the goulash over the rice noodles into a warm serving dish, sprinkled with the sliced green onions.

Per serving: Calories: 622 Protein: 42g Carbs: 82g Fiber: 9g Sugar: 9g Fat: 14g

Sweet Spiced Stove Top Moroccan Chicken

SERVES 2 / PREP TIME: 5 MINUTES / COOK TIME: 40 MINUTES

The maple syrup in this recipe is teamed with the Moroccan spices for a delectable chicken dish.

1 tbsp olive oil
4 (5 oz) skinless chicken breasts
1 tsp cumin
1 tsp ground ginger
1 tsp ground cumin
Peel from half a lemon, chopped
3 tsp chopped fresh cilantro
2 tsp chopped fresh parsley

1 (15 oz) can diced tomatoes
1 tbsp pure maple syrup
1 tbsp fresh lime juice to serve

1. Heat the olive oil in a heavy saucepan.
2. Add the chicken breasts and fry them for 1-2 minutes.
3. Add the ginger, and cumin for 2-3 minutes.
4. Add the lemon peel, cilantro, and parsley.
5. Next, add the tomatoes and the maple syrup to cover the chicken.
6. Bring to a boil.
7. Reduce the heat to medium, cover, and simmer on low heat for about 35 minutes.
8. Squeeze over the lime juice to serve.

Per serving: Calories: 275 Protein: 33g Carbs: 8g Fiber: 2g Sugar: 6g Fat: 12g

Potato and Paprika Chicken Potage

SERVES 8 / PREP TIME: 5 MINUTES / COOK TIME: 25 MINUTES

This hearty soup makes a good mid-week evening meal.

---

2 tbsp olive oil
8 (5 oz) boneless skinless chicken breasts, halved
8 medium white potatoes, peeled and cubed
1 tbsp tomato paste
2 tsp paprika
2 tbsp red wine vinegar
1/3 cup sherry

1 tbsp garlic infused oil
4 cups low FODMAP chicken stock
1 tbsp chopped green onions (green tips only)
A pinch of salt to taste
1 tsp dried oregano

---

1. Heat 1 tbsp oil in a large pot over medium heat.
2. Add the chicken to the pan.
3. Sauté for 4 minutes, or until golden.
4. Remove the chicken and set aside.
5. Add the potatoes and tomato paste to the pan and cook for 1 minute.
6. Stir in the paprika, vinegar, sherry, garlic oil, and stock.
7. Bring to a boil and allow the liquid to reduce for 2 minutes.
8. Return the chicken to the pan, cover, and simmer for 10 minutes.
9. Add the green onions.
10. Stir well and simmer the soup with the lid off for another 8 minutes, or until the sauce is thickened and the potatoes and chicken are cooked through.

Per serving: Calories: 407 Protein: 39g Carbs: 40g Fiber: 5g Sugar: 2g Fat: 10g

Sweet and Spiced North African Fish Stew

SERVES 4 / PREP TIME: 5 MINUTES / COOK TIME: 20 MINUTES

This light, tasty stew is ready in a flash!

---

1 tbsp olive oil
1 tsp ground ginger
1 tsp ground cumin
1 tsp turmeric
1 cinnamon stick
1 (15 oz) can diced tomatoes
1 tbsp green onions (green tips only), sliced
A pinch of pink Himalayan sea salt/sea salt

1 lb white cod, cut into chunks
2 tsp pure maple syrup
1 tbsp fresh cilantro leaves

---

1. Heat the olive oil in a stock pot over medium heat.
2. Add the ginger, cumin, turmeric, and cinnamon stick and cook for 2 minutes, stirring regularly.
3. Add the tomatoes, green onions, and salt.
4. Cook, stirring frequently, for 10 minutes.
5. Add the cod and simmer for five minutes, or until the fish is almost cooked through and tender.
6. Add the syrup and cook for 2-3 more minutes.
7. To serve, ladle the stew into bowls and garnish with fresh cilantro leaves.

Per serving: Calories: 132 Protein: 17g Carbs: 6g Fiber: 2g Sugar: 4g Fat: 4g

Savory Pumpkin and Spinach Stew

SERVES 4 / PREP TIME: 10 MINUTES / COOK TIME: 40 MINUTES

This light tomato-based stew makes a lovely vegetarian entrée.

---

2 tbsp coconut oil
1 tsp whole cumin seeds
1 (7 lb) pumpkin, peeled and cut into medium chunks
2 (15 oz) cans diced tomatoes
1 cup water
1 tbsp chopped scallions (green tips only)

2 cups fresh spinach, washed and roughly chopped
1 tbsp fresh parsley, chopped

---

1. Heat the oil in a stock pot with a lid over medium heat.
2. Stir in the cumin seeds until fragrant, about 1 minute.
3. Next add the pumpkin, tomatoes, and water.
4. Stir, cover, and bring to a boil.
5. Uncover the pot and let it simmer for 15 minutes.
6. Simmer for another 15 minutes, stirring frequently this time.
7. Next, stir in the scallions and spinach and continue to simmer for a further 8 minutes.
8. Serve piping hot and garnish with the chopped parsley.

Per serving: Calories: 159 Protein: 4g Carbs: 23g Fiber: 8g Sugar: 8g Fat: 8g

Zucchini and Spinach Soup

SERVES 4 / PREP TIME: 5 MINUTES / COOK TIME: 35 MINUTES

Fresh and tasty!

---

3 zucchinis, diced
2 medium carrots, diced
1 large white potato, diced
Water to cook the vegetables
1 cup fresh spinach
A pinch of salt to taste
1 tsp dried basil
1 tbsp olive oil

---

1. In a large saucepan, add the zucchini, carrots, and potato.
2. Pour in enough water to cover the vegetables.
3. Bring to a gentle boil and cook over medium heat for 30 minutes, or until the vegetables are mushy.
4. Allow to cool slightly.
5. Purée the soup in a blender or in the pot with a stick blender.
6. Season the soup with the salt and basil.
7. Stir in the spinach, cover, and simmer for 5 more minutes.
8. Just before serving, stir in the olive oil.

Per serving: Calories: 141 Protein: 4g Carbs: 24g Fiber: 5g Sugar: 6g Fat: 4g

Garbanzo Bean and Pepper Stew with Quinoa

SERVES 1 / PREP TIME: 5 MINUTES / COOK TIME: 30 MINUTES

Hearty and wholesome.

---

1 tbsp garlic-infused olive oil
1 large carrot, peeled and sliced
1 red bell pepper, seeded and chopped
1 large tomato, chopped
1/2 cup dry red wine
1 tsp paprika
A pinch cinnamon
1 tsp dried oregano
1/4 tsp salt

1/2 cup quinoa
1 cup water
1/2 cup canned garbanzo beans, drained and rinsed
1/4 cup sliced chives (green tips only)
1 tbsp fresh cilantro, chopped
1/2 tbsp fresh lemon juice

---

1. Heat the garlic oil in a large pot over medium-high heat.
2. Add the carrot, bell pepper, tomato, wine, paprika, cinnamon, oregano, and salt.
3. Bring all of this to a boil.
4. Once the mixture boils, reduce the heat to a simmer and cook, covered, for 15 minutes.
5. Meanwhile, in a small saucepan, bring the quinoa and water to a boil.
6. Once it is boiling, reduce the heat to low, cover, and cook for 15-20 minutes or until the water is mostly absorbed.
7. After the stew has been cooking for 15 minutes, add the garbanzo beans, chives, cilantro, and lemon juice.
8. Continue to simmer for 5-10 minutes or until thoroughly hot through.
9. Serve immediately.

Per serving: Calories: 399 Protein: 12g Carbs: 54g Fiber: 11g Sugar: 1g Fat: 11g

Spiced Chicken and Brown Rice Soup

SERVES 4 / PREP TIME: 10 MINUTES / COOK TIME: 50 MINUTES

If you like chicken and rice, you'll love this cinnamon and turmeric version!

---

4 (5 oz) boneless skinless chicken breasts
8 cups water
8 fresh thyme sprigs
1/2 tbsp turmeric
1/2 tsp ground cinnamon
1 large celery stalk with leaves, chopped
A pinch of salt to taste
1 tsp dried oregano

1/2 cup thinly sliced carrots
1 1/2 cups cooked brown rice

---

1. Add the chicken, water, 6 of the sprigs of thyme, turmeric, cinnamon, celery, and salt to a medium stock pot over high heat.
2. Bring the mixture to boil and lower to a rolling simmer for 20 minutes.
3. Check the chicken to ensure it is cooked throughout.
4. Add the carrots to the stock.
5. Turn the heat back on to high and boil for 5 minutes, or until the carrots are tender.
6. Add in the cooked rice and reduce the heat to a simmer.
7. Remove the sprigs of thyme with a slotted spoon.
8. Pour the soup in a large serving bowl and add fresh thyme as a garnish.

Hint: The chicken should be piping hot and completely white through the centre once cooked.

Per serving: Calories: 263 Protein: 34g Carbs: 19 g Fiber: 2g Sugar: 1g Fat: 4g

Hearty Turkey Chili

SERVES 4 / PREP TIME: 5 MINUTES / COOK TIME: 55 MINUTES

This chili is full of flavorful spices.

---

2 cups water
3/4 cup crushed tomatoes
2 tbsp garlic infused oil, divided
1 lb lean ground turkey
1 green bell pepper, seeded and diced
1 1/4 tsp ground cumin
A pinch of salt to taste
1 cup canned garbanzo beans, drained and rinsed

4 green onions (green tips only), diced

---

1. Bring the water to a boil in a pan over high heat.
2. Add the crushed tomatoes and 1 tbsp garlic-infused oil to the water.
3. Transfer this mixture to the bowl of a blender until smooth.
4. Meanwhile, add 1 tbsp garlic oil to a large Dutch oven or stock pot.
5. Add the turkey and cook for 20 minutes over medium heat.
6. Add the bell pepper and cook for 5 more minutes, or until the pepper is softened.
7. Add the cumin and salt to the pot.
8. Bring to a boil.
9. Then reduce the heat to medium-low and simmer for 30 minutes.
10. Add the green onions and stir before serving.

Per serving: Calories: 280 Protein: 30g Carbs: 18g Fiber: 5g Sugar: 5g Fat: 10g

SIDES, SALADS, SNACKS AND SAUCES

Baba Ganoush Dip

SERVES: 8 / PREP TIME: 15 MINUTES / COOK TIME: 45 MINUTES

You'll love this smoky dip with crudités!

---

1 medium eggplant (about 1 pound)
1 cup cooked or canned chickpeas, rinsed and drained
1 tbsp garlic infused oil
2 tbsp tahini paste

1/4 tsp salt
1/4 cup fresh lemon juice
1 tbsp finely chopped fresh cilantro

---

1. Preheat broiler to medium-low heat.
2. Prick the eggplant in several places with a fork and place on a baking sheet (whole).
3. Broil on the top shelf for 45 minutes, turning every 10 minutes or so, until eggplant is charred all over.
4. Remove and cover very loosely with foil to allow to sweat for 10 minutes.
5. When cool, remove the skin and transfer pulp to a blender or food processor. Add all remaining ingredients except cilantro and purée until very smooth.
6. Transfer to serving bowl and sprinkle with cilantro.

Hint: Drizzle a little olive oil over the dip just before serving for a little extra indulgence.

Per serving: Calories: 69 Protein: 2g Carbs: 8g Fiber: 2g Sugar: 2g Fat: 3g

Parsley and Cumin Lentils

SERVES: 2 / PREP TIME: 5 MINUTES / COOK TIME: 30 MINUTES

Lentils can be enjoyed in small quantities and are a great source of protein.

---

1 cup canned/dry red lentils
1 tbsp garlic infused oil
1 tbsp fresh parsley
1 tsp olive oil
1/2 tsp cumin

1/2 tsp turmeric
1/4 cup water

1 cup spinach, washed

---

1. If using dry lentils, soak in warm water overnight before using.
2. If using canned, simply drain before using.
3. Whisk together the garlic oil and parsley and place to one side.
4. Heat the olive oil in a small pan over medium heat and add the lentils.
5. Now sprinkle over the cumin and turmeric, pour in the water, cover and lower the heat.
6. Allow to steam for 20-30 minutes (keep an eye on the water to make sure the lentils don't burn).
7. When the water has been soaked up and the lentils are soft, remove and serve on a bed of spinach with a drizzle of the garlic and parsley dressing.

Per serving: Calories: 381 Protein: 25g Carbs: 56g Fiber: 22g Sugar: 5g Fat: 8g

Pineapple and Tomato Salsa

SERVES: 2 / PREP TIME: 5 MINUTES / COOK TIME: 30 MINUTES

So simple yet delicious.

---

4 ripe large tomatoes
1 tbsp fresh lime juice
1/4 cup pineapple, diced
A pinch of salt and pepper

---

1. Preheat broiler to low.
2. Slice the tomatoes in half and layer onto an oven sheet (skin side up).
3. Broil tomatoes for 7-8 minutes or until lightly chargrilled, turning to cook evenly on both sides.
4. Remove and allow to cool.
5. Once cool, dice the tomatoes with a sharp knife and transfer to a serving bowl.
6. Mix in the rest of the ingredients and enjoy with your favorite meat, fish or vegetable entrée.

Per serving: Calories: 61 Protein: 3g Carbs: 14g Fiber: 4g Sugar: 9g Fat: 1g

Homemade Ketchup

SERVING SIZE: 1 TBSP / PREP TIME: 5 MINUTES / COOK TIME: NA

A homemade version of the shop bought favorite.

---

12 oz tomato paste
½ cup brown sugar
2/3 cup water
4 tbsp white wine vinegar
½ tsp sea salt

---

1. Mix together all of the ingredients until the sugar is completely dissolved.
2. You can then refrigerate your ketchup for up to 3 to 4 weeks in an airtight container.

Please note this makes approx. 1 cup sauce and nutritional information is based on a serving size of 1 tbsp

Per serving: Calories: 88 Protein: 2g Carbs: 21g Fiber: 2g Sugar: 18g Fat: 0g

Strawberry Jam

SERVES: 4 / PREP TIME: 5 MINUTES / COOK TIME: 20 MINUTES

Make your own jam and enjoy on toast and crumpets!

---

2 cups strawberries, washed and sliced
1 tbsp stevia powder
1 tbsp fresh lemon juice

---

1. Combine all of the ingredients together over high heat in a small pan.
2. Bring your mixture to the boil then lower the heat and simmer, stirring occasionally with a wooden spoon for 5-10 minutes.
4. Reduce the heat down to low and then allow the mixture to simmer for a further 10 minutes.
5. Allow to cool, blend until smooth and then transfer to a Mason jar or airtight container.
6. You can then store the contents for up to 2-3 days in the fridge.

Top tip: wash out your old jam jars and save for future homemade jams and sauces. The seal will be broken so make sure you keep anything you store in the fridge only up to 2-3 days.

Per serving: Calories: 23 Protein: 0g Carbs: 6g Fiber: 1g Sugar: 4g Fat: 0g

Classic Pesto Spread

SERVES 4 / PREP TIME: 5 MINUTES / COOK TIME: NA

This fast and easy spread does wonders for any Italian entrée!

---

1 cup fresh basil, packed
1/4 cup pecan nuts
1/4 cup garlic-infused olive oil
1/4 cup feta cheese
1 tsp salt

---

1. Combine the basil and the pecan nuts in a food processor.
2. Pulse until coarsely chopped.
3. Slowly add the garlic-infused olive oil in a constant stream while the food processor is on.
4. Add the feta cheese and pulse again until well-blended and smooth.
5. Pulse in the salt.
6. Serve immediately, or store in an airtight container and refrigerate until you are ready to use it.

Hint: If freezing, transfer it to an air-tight container and drizzle some olive oil on top. It's also wise to eliminate the cheese initially and add it when you intend to use the pesto.

Per serving: Calories: 203 Protein: 3g Carbs: 2g Fiber: 0g Sugar: 1g Fat: 21g

Homemade Tasty BBQ Sauce

SERVES 6 / PREP TIME: 10 MINUTES / COOK TIME: 10 MINUTES

This delectable homemade BBQ will make you never want to buy it again!

2 tbsp potato starch
1/2 cup cold water
1/2 cup hot water
3 tbsp coconut sugar
1 cup red wine vinegar

1 tbsp garlic-infused olive oil
1 tsp salt
1/4 tsp asafoetida powder (garlic and onion replacement)
1/4 tsp liquid smoke

1. Mix the potato starch with the cold water and set aside.
2. In a sauce pan, combine the hot water and sugar, stirring until the sugar is dissolved.
3. Bring this to a boil and cook for 5 minutes.
4. Stir in the cornstarch and all remaining ingredients.
5. Mix well.
6. Bring to a boil, then reduce the heat and simmer, uncovered, for 5 minutes.
7. Remove from the heat and allow to cool to room temperature.
8. Use the sauce immediately or refrigerate in an airtight container up to 1 week.

Per serving: Calories: 69 Protein: 0g Carbs: 12g Sugar: 9g Fat: 2g

Cheesy Homemade Zucchini Chips

SERVES 4 / PREP TIME: 10 MINUTES / COOK TIME: 1 HOUR

This take on a popular healthy snack will have you making this recipe again and again!

---

2 medium zucchinis, very thinly sliced
2 tsp olive oil
1/2 tbsp hard parmesan cheese, freshly grated
1/4 tsp salt

---

1. Line a baking sheets with parchment paper.
2. Preheat the oven to 100 degrees, or its lowest setting.
3. Using a mandolin slicer set to 1/8-inch thickness, slice the zucchinis. Alternatively use a sharp knife and slice the zucchinis as thinly as possible.
4. Place the zucchini slices in a medium bowl and add the olive oil, parmesan cheese, and salt.
5. Toss the bowl to evenly coat each slice of zucchini.
6. Evenly space out the zucchini slices on the baking sheets so that none are overlapping.
7. Bake the zucchini at 100 degrees for 1 hour.
8. Store chips in an air-tight container.

Per serving: Calories: 40 Protein: 1g Carbs: 3g Fiber: 1g Sugar: 2g Fat: 3g

Pumpkin Spice Cookies

SERVES 12 COOKIES / PREP TIME: 10 MINUTES / COOK TIME: 10 MINUTES

These chocolate and pumpkin cookies are so soft, they're like little muffin bites!

1/2 cup melted coconut oil
1/2 cup coconut sugar
1 tsp vanilla extract
6 tbsp pumpkin purée
1 1/2 cups rice flour
1 tsp xanthan gum
1/4 tsp salt
1/2 tsp baking soda

1/4 tsp baking powder
1/2 cup cocoa powder

---

1. Preheat the oven to 350 degrees.
2. In a large bowl, mix together the coconut oil, coconut sugar, vanilla extract, and pumpkin purée until smooth.
3. Set this aside while mixing the flour.
4. In another bowl, whisk together the rice flour, xanthan gum, salt, baking soda, baking powder, and cocoa powder.
5. Gradually add the flour mixture to the wet ingredients until everything is combined.
6. Fold in the cocoa powder.
7. If your dough is too sticky to handle at this stage, cover and refrigerate it for at least 10 minutes.
8. Line a baking sheet with parchment paper or grease with a little coconut oil.
9. Roll out the dough into little balls about the size of a tablespoon.
10. Place them on the baking sheet.
11. Press down on each ball to flatten.
12. Bake the cookies for 8-10 minutes.
13. Leave to cool on the baking sheet for about 5 minutes before transferring them to a cooling rack.

Hint: The cooling process is vital as there is no egg in this recipe and they will crumble if you eat them hot.

Per serving: Calories: 192 Protein: 2g Carbs: 26g Sugar: 8g Fat: 10g

Homemade Rice Cakes

SERVES 2 (2 CAKES EACH) / PREP TIME: 5 MINUTES / COOK TIME: 20 MINUTES

Experiment with ingredients to create simply wonderful snacks!

¾ cup basmati rice, pre-boiled and
cooled
1 beef tomato, finely diced
1/4 cup goats cheese, crumbled
1 tbsp dried mixed herbs
3 egg whites, lightly beaten

---

1. Preheat oven to 400 degrees.
2. Line a muffin sheet with 4 muffin cups.
3. Mix the cooled rice, diced tomato, cheese, herbs, and egg whites in a mixing bowl until combined.
4. Then, spoon out your mixture into the muffin cases.
5. Bake the rice cakes for 15 to 20 minutes until golden in color and firm.
6. Allow to cool for 5 minutes and then use a knife to ease the edges out.
7. Let them cool for a few more minutes and then serve.

Per serving: Calories: 237 Protein: 15g Carbs: 21g Sugar: 3g Fat: 10g

Mini Chicken Quiches

SERVES 4 / PREP TIME: 5 MINUTES / COOK TIME: 20 MINUTES

Great for on the go lunches!

4 tbsp rice milk
2 tbsp rice flour
4 egg whites
A pinch of salt and pepper
½ red bell pepper, finely diced
1 scallion stem, finely diced (green tip only)

1 tsp dried thyme
1 cup diced skinless cooked chicken breasts

1. Preheat oven to 350 degrees.
2. Line a muffin sheet with 4 muffin cups.
3. Mix the rice milk and rice flour together in a mixing bowl.
4. Then, whisk in the egg whites along with a pinch of salt and pepper.
5. Whisk until smooth.
6. Mix in the rest of the ingredients.
7. Pour the mixture into the cases evenly, leaving 1/2 cm gap at the top.
8. Bake for 15-20 minutes or until eggs are firm.
9. Remove from the oven and allow to cool before popping them out of their cases (or leave them in and pop them in a lunch box for later!)

Per serving: Calories: 101 Protein: 15g Carbs: 6gSugar: 2g Fat: 2g

Cucumber and Goats Cheese Rolls

SERVES 6 / PREP TIME: 10 MINUTES / COOK TIME: NA

Quick and healthy snacks.

---

1 large cucumber
3/4 cup soft goats cheese, crumbled
2 tsp garlic infused oil
2 tsp fresh dill, chopped
1/2 tsp dried oregano
1 green onion, sliced (green tips only)
A pinch of sea salt
6 toothpicks

---

1. Wash the cucumber.
2. Cut the cucumber by trimming the ends and cutting the flesh lengthwise (aim for 6 slices).
3. In a small bowl, toss the goats cheese with the garlic infused oil, the dill, and the oregano.
4. Place 1 tbsp the cheese mixture at the end of each cucumber slice.
5. Garnish the cheese with the green onion slices and the salt.
6. Roll each slice up and pierce it with a toothpick to hold it together.
7. Serve the cucumber roll ups on a plate for a light snack.

Per serving: Calories: 82 Protein: 4g Carbs: 1g Fiber: 0g Sugar: 1g Fat: 7g

Zesty Lime Sweet Potato Fries

SERVES 2 / PREP TIME: 10 MINUTES / COOK TIME: 45 MINUTES

The lime in this recipe enhances these sweet potatoes and gives them a unique flavor.

1 medium sweet potato
1 1/2 tbsp fresh lime juice
2 tsp lime zest
1 tbsp coconut oil, melted
1/2 tsp paprika
A pinch of salt to taste

1. Preheat the oven to 400 degrees.
2. Slice the sweet potato into fries, (approx. 1/2 inch by 3 inch strips).
3. Add the potato slices to a medium bowl and drizzle them with the lime juice, zest, oil, paprika, and salt.
4. Place the potatoes on a lightly oiled cookie sheet or one lined with parchment paper.
5. Bake for 35-45 minutes, or until crisp.

Hint: Soften the sweet potato before slicing it by cooking it in the microwave for about 3-4 minutes, being sure to pierce the skin with a fork or knife several times before cooking. Let the potato cool for 30 minutes so you can handle it.

Per serving: Calories: 119 Protein: 1 g Carbs: 14g Fiber: 2g Sugar: 3g Fat: 7g

Quick Tossed Tomatoes and Basil

SERVES 2 / PREP TIME: 5 MINUTES / COOK TIME: NA

This fast and easy salad makes eating healthy a breeze!

---

2 tbsp garlic-infused olive oil
1/4 cup chopped fresh basil
1/2 cup diced Roma tomatoes
A pinch of salt to taste
1/2 tsp dried oregano

---

1. Toss together the salad ingredients in a salad bowl and serve immediately.
2. If preparing for later on, leave the oil until the last minute.

Per serving: Calories: 147 Protein: 1g Carbs: 3g Fiber: 1g Sugar: 1g Fat: 15g

Easy Homemade Oven Fries

SERVES 3 / PREP TIME: 5 MINUTES / COOK TIME: 25 MINUTES

These simple baked potato fries make a great snack or side to any entrée!

---

6 small red potatoes, washed
1 tbsp garlic infused oil
1 tbsp chopped fresh rosemary
1 tsp paprika
A pinch of salt and pepper to taste

---

1. Preheat the oven to 400 degrees.
2. Slice the potatoes into wedges and place them onto a cookie sheet.
3. Drizzle them evenly with the garlic oil.
4. Sprinkle the rosemary, paprika, salt, and pepper over the potatoes.
5. Bake for 25 minutes.
6. Turn potatoes halfway through baking to cook them evenly.
7. Remove from the oven and serve.

Per serving: Calories: 235 Protein: 4g Carbs: 37g Fiber: 4g Sugar: 3g Fat: 9g

Mediterranean Quinoa and Sweet Potato Salad

SERVES 4 / PREP TIME: 5 MINUTES / COOK TIME: 25 MINUTES

Crumbled feta with sweet potato salad.

---

1 sweet potato
1 tbsp olive oil
1/2 cup red quinoa
1 cup water
A pinch of salt to taste
1 cup fresh spinach
1/4 cup feta cheese, crumbled

3 tbsp olive oil
1 tbsp balsamic vinegar
1 dash dried oregano
A pinch of salt to taste

---

1. Preheat the oven to 400 degrees.
2. Cut the sweet potato into cubes and place onto a baking sheet.
3. Drizzle with the olive oil and place the sheet in the oven for 20-25 minutes.
4. Meanwhile, rinse the quinoa in cold water.
5. Combine with the cup of water and salt in a saucepan and bring to a boil.
6. Turn the heat down to medium and simmer for 15 minutes, or until all the water is absorbed.
7. Turn off the heat and cover for 5 minutes.
8. Fluff the quinoa with a fork and set it aside to cool.
9. Now toss together the spinach and feta cheese in a medium bowl.
10. Gently add the cooled sweet potatoes and quinoa to the spinach and feta cheese.
11. Make the dressing by mixing together the rest of the ingredients.
12. Drizzle the dressing over the bowl of quinoa and sweet potato salad.
13. Serve with salad tongs.

Per serving: Calories: 254 Protein: 5g Carbs: 21g Fiber: 3g Sugar: 3g Fat: 17g

Zesty Kale Salad

SERVES 4 / PREP TIME: 5 MINUTES / COOK TIME: 20 MINUTES

This lemony kale salad tossed with quinoa makes a great lunch!

1/2 cup quinoa, rinsed
1 cup boiling water
1/4 cup olive oil
1/4 cup apple cider vinegar
1 lemon, juice and zest
1 tbsp coconut sugar
A pinch of salt and pepper to taste
2 cups chopped kale, de-stemmed

1/2 cup red grapes, seedless and halved
1/4 cup crumbled feta cheese

---

1. Bring the quinoa and water to the boil in a saucepan.
2. Lower the heat to medium, cover and simmer for 15 minutes.
3. Meanwhile, make the vinaigrette - whisk together the olive oil, apple cider vinegar, lemon juice, lemon zest, sugar, salt, and pepper in a small bowl.
4. Set aside the vinaigrette.
5. Drain the quinoa once most of the water has been absorbed in the pan.
6. To assemble the salad, place the kale in a large bowl.
7. Top it with the quinoa, grapes, and feta cheese.
8. Pour the dressing on top of the salad and gently toss to combine.
9. Serve immediately.

Per serving: Calories: 225 Protein: 4g Carbs: 16g Fiber: 2g Sugar: 2g Fat: 16g

Gluten Free Chicken Vermicelli and Tomato Salad

SERVES 4 / PREP TIME: 10 MINUTES / COOK TIME: NA

A delicious and light Summer salad.

½ red bell pepper, diced
4 large tomatoes, sliced
1 cup romaine lettuce, chopped
2 (5 oz) cooked chicken breasts, sliced
2 tbsp low FODMAP pesto
2 tbsp lactose free sour cream (optional)
2 cups rice vermicelli, cooked according to package

1 tbsp fresh basil, torn
1 tbsp olive oil
A pinch of salt to taste

---

1. For the salad, mix the red pepper with the tomatoes, lettuce, and chicken in a medium bowl.
2. In a separate bowl, mix the pesto and the lactose free sour cream.
3. Stir the cooked vermicelli into the pesto mix.
4. Lay the noodles onto plates.
5. Top with a portion of the salad.
6. Drizzle the salad with the olive oil and sprinkle on the basil, salt, and pepper.

Hint: Use the pesto recipe earlier in this section.

Per serving: Calories: 298 Protein: 25g Carbs: 26g Sugar: 4g Fat: 10g

Tropical Rice

SERVES 5 / PREP TIME: 15 MINUTES / COOK TIME: 2 HOURS SLOW COOKER

This tastes amazing with curries, grilled meats and fish.

---

2 cups jasmine rice
4 cups water
1 cup canned pineapple, diced
1 lime, juice
1 crushed lemongrass stem

---

1. Add the rice, water, pineapple, lime juice, and lemongrass into the slow cooker.
2. Set the slow cooker to HIGH for 2 hours or LOW for 4-5 hours.
3. Remove the lemongrass before serving.

Per serving: Calories: 247 Protein: 3g Carbs: 22g Sugar: 4g Fat: 17g

DRINKS AND DESSERTS

Strawberry and Carob Shake

SERVES 1 / PREP TIME: 5 MINUTES / COOK TIME: NA

Think chocolate covered strawberries in a glass!

1/2 cup strawberries, washed and
sliced
1 pasteurised egg white
1/4 cup vanilla rice milk
1 tbsp carob powder

---

1. Combine ingredients in a blender or smoothie maker until smooth.
2. Pour over ice if desired.

Per serving: Calories: 163 Protein: 7g Carbs: 36g Sugar: 20g Fat: 1g

Moroccan Mint Tea

SERVES 6 / PREP TIME: 5 MINUTES / COOK TIME: NA

Mint tea is enjoyed as a refreshing drink in Morocco and is packed with goodness.

---

2 cups packed fresh mint leaves
6 cups boiling water
4 slices lemon

---

1. Place all ingredients in a teapot, and stir.
2. Let steep for 4 minutes.
3. Stir well and add maple syrup if desired.
4. Serve hot or chilled.

Per serving (without maple syrup): Calories: 0 Protein: 0g Carbs: 0 Sugar: 0g Fat: 0g

Chocolate Banana Smoothie

SERVES 1 / PREP TIME: 5 MINUTES / COOK TIME: NA

A mood boosting smoothie for breakfast or as a dessert.

1/2 banana, peeled and sliced
1/2 cup rice milk
1 tbsp baking cocoa powder,
unsweetened
1 tsp vanilla extract
Ice cubes or crushed ice
1 tbsp pure maple syrup (optional)

---

1. Place all of the ingredients into a blender.
2. Blend until smooth, making sure no ice chunks remain.
3. Transfer to a serving glass and drink at once.

Per serving: Calories: 175 Protein: 2g Carbs: 39g Fiber: 4g Sugar: 29g Fat: 2g

Fruity Mint Virgin Cocktail

SERVES 1 / PREP TIME: 5 MINUTES / COOK TIME: NA

This sweet drink is a refreshing choice on a hot afternoon.

---

1 cup cranberry juice, no sugar added
½ cup frozen raspberries
2 fresh mint sprigs, to serve

---

1. Place all the ingredients into a blender.
2. Pulse until the consistency is smooth.
3. Pour the cocktail into a glass of your choice.
4. Serve topped with fresh mint.

Per serving: Calories: 149 Protein: 2g Carbs: 38g Fiber: 4g Sugar: 29g Fat: 1g

Blueberry Vanilla Milkshake

SERVES 1 / PREP TIME: 10 MINUTES / COOK TIME: NA

This scrumptious milkshake is both healthy and satisfying.

½ cup organic blueberries
1 tsp vanilla extract
1 cup almond milk
1 handful crushed ice

1. In a blender, pulse together the blueberries, vanilla extract, almond milk, and ice.
2. Pour the shake into a milkshake glass.

Per serving: Calories: 147 Protein: 2g Carbs: 27g Fiber: 3g Sugar: 23g Fat: 3g

Tropical Fruit Shake

SERVES 4 / PREP TIME: 10 MINUTES / COOK TIME: NA

Satisfy your sweet tooth with this tasty shake!

---

1 cup crushed ice
½ cup almond/cashew milk
1/2 ripe banana, cut into chunks
3 whole strawberries, stems removed
and halved
¼ cup organic raspberries, plus extra
to garnish

---

1. Add the ice to the blender and crush.
2. Now add the rest of the ingredients to the blender.
3. Blend the mixture for approximately 1 minute.
4. Pour into glasses to serve and add one or two raspberries as garnish.

Per serving: Calories: 127 Protein: 2g Carbs: 28g Fiber: 5g Sugar: 18g Fat: 2g

Raspberry and Almond Cake

SERVES 8 / PREP TIME: 20 MINUTES/ COOK TIME: 30 MINUTES

Raspberries and almonds blend perfectly in this divine cake recipe.

---

2 cups fresh raspberries
1/2 cup almonds, finely ground
1/4 cup packed brown sugar
8 plus 1 tbsp rice flour
3 large egg whites
1/8 teaspoon salt

8 tbsp canola oil
1 tsp vanilla extract
1/2 tsp almond extract
1 tsp granulated sugar

---

1. Preheat oven to 375 degrees.
2. Add fresh raspberries to a small saucepan with 1 tbsp water over high heat.
3. Bring to a boil and reduce the heat, simmering until just soft (5 minutes).
4. Spray a 5 inch non-stick spring-form pan with cooking oil and set aside.
5. In a medium bowl whisk together ground almonds, brown sugar, and 8 tbsp rice flour until well combined.
6. In a separate (large) bowl beat the egg whites with the salt to form stiff peaks and then fold in the nut mixture from earlier.
7. Now fold in the oil, vanilla extract, and almond extract, and spread the batter in the pan.
8. Spread the raspberries evenly over the batter and sprinkle with granulated sugar.
9. Bake for 20-30 minutes or until a knife comes out clean from the center.
10. Remove and cool on a wired rack.
11. Portion up and serve.

Per serving: Calories: 281 Protein: 5g Carbs: 23g Fiber: 4g Sugar: 9 g Fat: 20g

Chocolate Pudding

SERVES 3 / PREP TIME: 10 MINUTES/ COOK TIME: 10 MINUTES

Satisfy your chocolate cravings with this dessert.

---

3 tbsp granulated sugar
1/4 cup unsweetened cocoa powder
3 tbsp cornstarch (or potato starch)
3 large pasteurised egg whites
3 cups vanilla rice milk
3 tbsp maple syrup
1/2 tbsp vanilla extract

---

1. Whisk together the sugar, cocoa powder, and cornstarch in a large heatproof glass bowl.
2. In a separate small bowl beat the egg whites until lightly frothy and set aside.
3. Gradually whisk the rice milk and maple syrup into the cocoa powder mix until well blended.
4. Bring a pan of water to the boil over high heat and place the glass bowl over the top, whilst whisking constantly until the mixture reaches a boil.
5. Continue whisking for one more minute then remove from heat.
6. Carefully whisk several large spoonfuls of hot pudding into the egg whites to temper.
7. Add the egg mixture back to the glass bowl and whisk well to thoroughly blend.
8. Return the pan to the heat and whisk constantly for one minute until mixture thickens.
9. Remove from heat and pour into three serving glasses.
10. Chill until cold.

Per serving: Calories: 243 Protein: 11g Carbs: 43g Fiber: 3g Sugar: 36 g Fat: 5g

Fat-Free Ginger Maple Cookies

SERVES 12 COOKIES / PREP TIME: 10 MINUTES / COOK TIME: 10 MINUTES

These easy gluten free cookies might just become your new favorite snack!

---

1 cup rice flour
½ tsp baking soda
¼ tsp salt
1/4 tsp ground ginger
½ cup pure maple syrup
2 egg whites

---

1. Preheat the oven to 350 degrees.
2. Sift the dry ingredients together in a bowl and set aside.
3. In a large bowl, whisk together the maple syrup and egg whites until combined.
4. Gradually, add the dry ingredients to this bowl.
5. Mix the batter together with a wooden spoon.
6. Now place tablespoons of dough onto a cookie sheet lined with parchment paper.
7. Use a fork to press each cookie ball down, forming a cross pattern on each.
8. Place the sheet in the oven for 5-10 minutes.

Per serving: Calories: 86 Protein: 1g Carbs: 19g Fiber: 0g Sugar: 9g Fat: 0g

Cranberry Orange Oatmeal Cookies

SERVES 12 COOKIES / PREP TIME:2 HOURS COOLING/ COOK TIME: 10 MINUTES

The zest of the orange in this recipe cuts through the sweet and sour cranberries.

---

1 cup oat flour
1/2 cup cornmeal
1/2 tsp baking powder
1 overripe banana, mashed
1/4 cup coconut sugar
1 large egg white
1 tsp vanilla extract

1/2 tsp ground cloves
1 tsp orange zest
1/4 cup organic cranberries, finely chopped

---

1. In a medium bowl, mix together the oat flour, cornmeal, and baking powder.
2. In another bowl, beat the banana and sugar until creamy.
3. Add in the egg white, vanilla extract, and ground cloves until blended.
4. Gradually add the dry ingredients to the wet until combined.
5. Fold in the orange zest and cranberries and mix into a dough.
6. Roll the dough out onto parchment paper and form it into a 2-inch diameter roll.
7. Place the roll of dough in the refrigerator until it is firm, or about 2 hours.
8. When ready to bake, preheat the oven to 350 degrees.
9. Slice the dough into 1/4 inch slices.
10. Place the cookies on a baking sheet lined with parchment paper.
11. Bake for about 10 minutes.
12. Let the cookies cool before serving.

Hint: The 2-inch dough roll will be about 14 inches long with flat edges, so it will have more of a square shape.

Per serving: Calories: 118 Protein: 3g Carbs: 24g Sugar: 6g Fat: 1g

Classic Blueberry Muffins

SERVES 4 / PREP TIME: 5 MINUTES / COOK TIME: 20 MINUTES

These yummy muffins are amazing with a cup of tea or coffee.

1 ripe mashed banana
1/2 cup coconut sugar
3 egg whites
2 cups gluten-free all purpose baking flour
¼ cup blueberries

¼ cup unsweetened coconut flakes
1/2 cup cashew milk
1 tsp vanilla extract

1. Preheat the oven to 350 degrees.
2. Mix the banana and the sugar together until a creamy paste is formed.
3. Now add in the egg whites and whisk until light and fluffy.
4. Fold in the flour using a wooden spoon or spatula.
5. Once the flour is completely mixed in, add the blueberries and most of the coconut flakes.
6. Add the milk slowly to ensure the mixture stays moist.
7. Spoon the mixture into a muffin pan lined with muffin papers.
8. Sprinkle the remaining coconut on top of the muffins.
9. Place in the oven for 20 minutes.
10. Once baked, the muffins should be springy to the touch.
11. When they are done, leave them to cool for 10 minutes and then enjoy!

Per serving: Calories: 116 Protein: 2g Carbs: 25g Sugar: 10g Fat: 1g

Chocolatey Coconut Meringues

SERVES 16 MERINGUES / PREP TIME: 10 MINUTES / COOK TIME: 8 MINUTES

These little bite-size chocolate meringues will melt in your mouth!

---

3 egg whites
3/4 cup coconut sugar, finely ground in
spice or coffee grinder
3/4 cup unsweetened cocoa powder
¼ cup unsweetened coconut flakes
1/2 tsp vanilla extract
A pinch of sea salt

---

1. Preheat the oven to 350 degrees.
2. Line a cookie sheet with parchment paper.
3. In a medium bowl, whisk the egg whites until they form fluffy soft peaks.
4. Gradually whisk in the sugar, cocoa powder, coconut, vanilla, and sea salt.
5. Drop the meringues by the teaspoonful onto the baking sheets.
6. Try to form approx. 15 small cookies.
7. Bake for 8 minutes. They should be a little puffed up with a slight crust on top of each cookie.
8. Allow to cool and then enjoy.

Per serving: Calories: 53 Protein: 2g Carbs: 12g Sugar: 9g Fat: 1g

Old Fashioned Raspberry Pancakes

SERVES 4 / PREP TIME: 5 MINUTES / COOK TIME: 15 MINUTES

These out flour pancakes might shock you with how delicious they are!

1/2 cup pure maple syrup
1 cup fresh or frozen raspberries
1 cup old fashioned rolled oats (gluten-free)
¼ tsp sea salt

1 tsp baking powder
1/2 cup cashew milk
1 egg white
1 tsp vanilla extract
1 tsp coconut oil

---

1. Warm the maple syrup and raspberries in a small saucepan over medium heat, stirring frequently, until the raspberries have thawed (if using frozen), about 3 minutes.
2. Take the pan off the heat and set aside.
3. Now place the oats and salt in a blender or a food processor and pulse until the consistency is that of coarse flour.
4. Pour this into a bowl and stir in the salt, and baking powder.
5. In a measuring jar, whisk together the cashew milk, egg white, and vanilla.
6. Then stir this wet mixture into the ground oats until thoroughly combined. (If the batter thickens too much, add more milk. Do not let this batter rest, as it will thicken quickly.)
7. Pour half the oil onto a smooth, non-stick griddle.
8. Put the griddle on medium heat and, when hot, add the batter.
9. Use a 1/4 cup measure to do this, but only fill it two-thirds full.
10. Cook about 4 pancakes at a time.
11. Cook for 2 minutes on both sides.
12. When you've cooked the first batch, pile them on a plate and cover with a clean tea towel.
13. Oil the pan again and continue cooking.
14. Serve immediately with the warm raspberry maple syrup poured on top.

Per serving: Calories: 218 Protein: 4g Carbs: 46g Sugar: 29g Fat: 3g

Gluten Free Chocolate Cake

SERVES 8 / PREP TIME: 10 MINUTES / COOK TIME: 45 MINUTES

You can still indulge once in a while!

1/2 cup unsweetened cocoa powder, sifted
1/2 cup boiling water
2 tsp vanilla extract
Gluten-free all purpose baking flour (double the volume of egg whites once measured)
½ tsp baking soda
1/4 tsp ground cinnamon

A pinch of salt
3/4 cup coconut sugar
1/2 cup coconut oil, plus extra for greasing
4 egg whites

1. Preheat the oven to 325 degrees.
2. Grease a 9-inch spring form cake pan with a little oil or line with parchment paper.
3. Sift the cocoa powder into a bowl and whisk in the boiling water until you have a smooth but still runny paste.
4. Whisk in the vanilla extract, then set aside to cool.
5. In another small bowl, combine the flour with the baking soda, cinnamon, cayenne, and a pinch of salt.
6. Beat the coconut sugar, coconut oil, and egg whites together in an electric mixer vigorously for about 3 minutes, or until it reaches a thick cream-like consistency.
7. Turn the speed down a little and pour in the cocoa mixture, beating as you go.
8. When it is all mixed, you can slowly pour in the flour mixture.
9. Pour this dark, liquid batter into the prepared pan.
10. Bake for 40-45 minutes, or until the sides are set. A toothpick should come out clean but with a few crumbs clinging to it.
11. Let it cool for 10 minutes on a wire rack.
12. Then scrape the sides of the cake with a butter knife and spring it out of the pan.
13. Serve either warm or cool.

Per serving: Calories: 258 Protein: 4g Carbs: 33g Sugar: 18g Fat: 15g

Minty Lime Sorbet

SERVES 4 / PREP TIME: 20 MINUTES / CHILLING TIME: 4 HOURS

A refreshing dessert.

¼ cup coconut sugar
2 cups boiling water
8 limes, juice
4 limes, zest
20 fresh mint leaves, minced
A pinch of sea salt
1 cup water

---

1. Make the sugar syrup by stirring the sugar in 2 cups boiling water until the sugar dissolves, about 5 minutes.
2. Set aside to cool.
3. Once cool, combine the syrup with the lime juice, zest, mint leaves, sea salt, and water.
4. Pour this mixture into a flat freezer-safe container (with a lid) and place it in the fridge for 30 minutes.
5. After it is thoroughly chilled, transfer to the freezer.
6. After about 45 minutes, take out and churn the sorbet with a fork, evening out what has started to freeze.
7. Return the sorbet to the freezer.
8. Repeat the churning every 45 minutes for at least 3-4 hours.

Per serving: Calories: 66 Protein: 0g Carbs: 19g Sugar: 14g Fat: 0g

Simple Orange-Pineapple Sorbet

SERVES 8 / PREP TIME: 5 MINUTES / CHILLING TIME: 4 HOURS

This 3-ingredient sorbet is so easy, you'll wonder why you haven't been making your own sorbet all along!

---

1 small pineapple, peeled, cored, and cubed
2 tbsp fresh orange juice
1 cup plus 2 tbsp coconut sugar
1 sprig fresh mint to serve

---

1. Place the pineapple and orange juice in a food processor.
2. Process until smooth.
3. Add the sugar and process for 1 minute, or until the sugar dissolves.
4. Pour this mixture into a flat freezer-safe container (with a lid) and place it in the fridge for 30 minutes.
5. After it is thoroughly chilled, transfer to the freezer.
6. After about 45 minutes, take out and churn the sorbet with a fork, evening out what has started to freeze.
7. Return the sorbet to the freezer.
8. Repeat the churning every 45 minutes for at least 3-4 hours.
9. To serve, garnish each dish with a mint leaf.

Per serving: Calories: 118 Protein: 0g Carbs: 27g Sugar: 27g Fat: 0g

Raspberry and Passion Fruit Sorbet

SERVES 8 / PREP TIME: 20 MINUTES / CHILLING TIME: 4 HOURS

This brightly flavored sorbet can easily be churned in an ice cream maker.

---

4 cups raspberries, fresh or frozen
1 cup passion-fruit juice
3/4 to 1 cup coconut sugar
A pinch of sea salt
3 tbsp lemon juice

---

1. Place the raspberries, passion-fruit juice, 3/4 cup coconut sugar, salt, and lemon juice into a blender.
2. Purée everything until it is very well blended.
3. Taste the mixture for tartness, and add more sugar if necessary, blending well.
4. Strain the mixture through a fine mesh sieve to remove the raspberry seeds.
5. Chill the mixture if it's not already cold.
6. Pour the mixture into an ice cream maker and freeze according to the directions.
7. After churning, place the sorbet in the freezer for 2-3 hours to finish freezing completely.
8. If not using an ice cream maker, pour the ingredients into a container and place it in the freezer for 30 minutes. Remove and stir it well with a fork.
9. Continue to freeze the mixture, stirring well every half hour for 4 hours until the sorbet is frozen to the desired texture.

Per serving: Calories: 141 Protein: 1g Carbs: 36g Sugar: 31g Fat: 1g

Simple Lemon Crépes

SERVES 4 / PREP TIME: 10 MINUTES / COOK TIME: 5-10 MINUTES

All you need is a little lemon juice to make these crépes fabulous!

---

1 cup rice flour, sifted
A pinch of salt
2 egg whites
1 dash vanilla extract
1 cup unsweetened light coconut milk
1 tbsp coconut oil

---

1. Sift the rice flour, and salt into a large mixing bowl.
2. Make a well in the centre of the flour and add the egg whites.
3. Begin whisking the egg whites into the flour.
4. Next gradually whisk in the vanilla extract and the coconut milk.
5. When all the liquid has been added, whisk until the batter is smooth and the consistency of thin cream.
6. Meanwhile, heat the coconut oil in a non-stick round skillet or crépe maker until it hot.
7. Turn the heat down to medium.
8. Spoon out two tablespoons of batter into the skillet.
9. As soon as the batter hits the hot skillet, tip it around from side to side to coat the skillet.
10. Cook on each side for about 30 seconds. Lift the edge with a butter knife to see if the bottom is golden brown before turning.
11. Flip the crépe over with a spatula, cook for 30 seconds, and slide onto a plate.
12. Stack the crépes between sheets of parchment paper as you make them.
13. Keep them warm by placing the pancake platter on top of a bowl filled with boiling water.
14. To serve, sprinkle each crépe with freshly squeezed lemon juice and coconut sugar.
15. Fold them in half, then in half again to form triangles. You may also simply roll them up.

Per serving: Calories: 183 Protein: 4g Carbs: 25g Sugar: 1g Fat: 8g

Gluten Free Glazed Lemon Donuts

SERVES 4 / PREP TIME: 30 MINUTES / COOK TIME: 20 MINUTES

These baked gluten free donuts can compete with store-bought ones any day!

1/3 cup coconut sugar	1/4 cup golden flax meal
2 tbsp coconut oil	1 tsp baking powder
3 egg whites	½ tsp salt
1/2 cup plain coconut milk yogurt	1 cup coconut sugar, finely ground in a
1 tsp lemon zest	spice or coffee grinder
1 tsp vanilla extract	2 tbsp lemon juice
½ cup rice flour	1 tbsp plain coconut milk yogurt
1/3 cup tapioca starch	1 tbsp lemon zest

1. Preheat the oven to 325 degrees.
2. In a large bowl, whisk the coconut sugar with the coconut oil for 2 minutes. (You may need to melt the coconut oil with the palms of your hands to whisk easier).
3. Add in the egg whites and beat the mixture until the batter starts to bubble.
4. Add in the yogurt, lemon zest, and vanilla extract and combine.
5. In another bowl, combine the rice flour, tapioca starch, flax meal, baking powder, and salt.
6. Slowly add this to the batter, beating until completely blended.
7. Spoon the batter into a donut pan or donut molds and bake for 15-20 minutes, or until golden.
8. Remove from the oven and leave to cool for 10 minutes before popping the donuts out of their molds.
9. For the lemon glaze, whisk together the ground sugar and lemon juice until smooth.
10. Add in the yogurt and whisk well.
11. Dip each donut into the glaze and sprinkle them with lemon zest to serve.

Per serving: Calories: 479 Protein: 5g Carbs: 93g Sugar: 67g Fat: 10g

Pina Colada Sorbet

SERVES 2 / PREP TIME: 4 HOURS FREEZING / COOK TIME: NA

A tropical cocktail-inspired dessert.

1 cup canned pineapple, diced
1 cup almond milk
1/4 cup desiccated coconut,
unsweetened
2 sprigs fresh mint

1. Blend the pineapple with the almond milk and coconut until smooth.
2. Pour into a plastic container and cover.
3. Place in the freezer for 2 hours.
4. Stir and replace for another 2 hours. Repeat if not yet set.
5. When set, serve immediately in a tall glass with a sprig of fresh mint.

Per serving: Calories: 88 Protein: 1g Carbs: 16g Sugar: 13g Fat: 3g

Orange Cranberry Cookies

SERVES 6 / PREP TIME: 2 HOURS COOLING / COOK TIME: 10 MINUTES

Treat yourself!

½ tsp baking powder
1 cup rice flour
¼ cup caster sugar
1 small mashed banana (very ripe)
1 tsp vanilla extract
2 egg whites
¼ cup organic cranberries, chopped
1 orange, juice and zest

---

1. Mix together the baking powder, rice flour and sugar in a large bowl.
2. Use another bowl to beat together the sugar and banana until the consistency is creamy.
3. Then add the vanilla and egg whites into the bowl with the banana and mix well.
4. Now fold the wet ingredients into the dry ingredients.
5. Fold in the cranberries and orange juice and zest and mix to dough consistency.
6. Use your hands to form a dough ball and wrap in plastic wrap.
7. Let the dough chill in the refrigerator for about 2 hours until firm.
8. Then, roll out the dough onto parchment paper and use cookie cutters to cut out your cookies, collecting the leftover dough and rolling out once more to cut as many cookies as you can.
9. Preheat your oven to 350 degrees when ready to cook.
10. Bake the cookies for 10 minutes and then allow to cool before serving.

Per serving: Calories: 159 Protein: 3g Carbs: 36g Sugar: 12g Fat: 0g

No Bake Lemon Raspberry Cheesecake with Gingersnap Crusts

SERVES 6 / PREP TIME: 20 MINUTES / CHILL TIME: 3 HOURS

Talk about the perfect balance of easy and delicious!

---

15 gluten free ginger snap cookies
1/3 cup coconut oil + extra for greasing
5 oz lactose free cream cheese
2 tbsp pure maple syrup
1 tsp vanilla extract
1/2 lemon, juiced
3/4 cup organic raspberries

---

1. To make the crust, gently pulse the ginger snaps and coconut oil in a food processor until the mixture has the consistency of sand.
2. Spread this mixture into a spring form pan, pie pan, or 8x8 baking dish greased generously with coconut oil.
3. Press the mixture down, smoothing with the back of a spoon until the crust is flat and even.
4. Put the pan in the fridge while you make the cheesecake layer.
5. Add the rest of the ingredients except the raspberries to the food processor and pulse until the mixture is smooth and creamy.
6. Mix in the raspberries by hand and set the processor bowl to the side.
7. Next, remove the crust from the fridge.
8. Spread the cheesecake filling evenly on top of the crust.
9. Cover the cheesecake with plastic wrap.
10. Return the pan to the fridge to set for 3 hours.
11. Remove the cheesecake from the fridge 10 minutes before serving.
12. Slice it into 12 bars and enjoy.

Per serving: Calories: 286 Protein: 3g Carbs: 23g Sugar: 15g Fat: 23g

Blueberry Rice Pudding

SERVES 6 / PREP TIME: 10 MINUTES / COOK TIME: 1.5 HOURS SLOW COOKER

Tastes great with blueberries or any low FODMAP fruit of your choice.

---

2 cups cooked white rice
1 tsp vanilla extract
4 cups almond milk
Maple syrup, to taste
1 cup blueberries

---

1. Stir the cooked rice, vanilla extract and almond milk into the slow cooker pot.
2. Set the slow cooker on HIGH for 1 1/2 hours.
3. To serve, stir in a little maple syrup with the blueberries.

Per serving (without maple syrup): Calories: 249 Protein: 3g Carbs: 44g Fiber: 2g
Sugar: 19g Fat: 3g

Slow-Cooked Fruit Crumble

SERVES 6 / PREP TIME: 10 MINUTES / COOK TIME: 2-3 HOURS SLOW COOKER

A home-cooked favorite.

---

3 cups sliced strawberries
2 cups sliced banana
1 tbsp grated lemon zest
1 cup gluten-free oats
¼ tsp ground cinnamon

---

1. Mix the strawberries, banana, and lemon zest, and place them in the slow cooker.
2. Mix the oats with the ground cinnamon, and top over the fruits.
3. Set the slow cooker to HIGH for 2-3 hours or until crumble is golden brown.

Per serving: Calories: 96 Protein: 3g Carbs: 20g Sugar: 7g Fat: 1g

Old-Fashioned Blueberry Crumble

SERVES 4 / PREP TIME: 15 MINUTES / COOK TIME: 40 MINUTES

Delicious blueberries simmer under a layer of sweet oats in this gluten free dessert.

2 1/4 cups organic blueberries
2 tbsp water
1 tbsp potato starch
3 tbsp coconut oil, melted
2/3 cup old fashioned rolled oats (gluten-free)
3 tbsp fresh ground oat flour

A pinch of salt
1 dash vanilla extract
2 tbsp pure maple syrup

1. Heat the oven to 350 degrees.
2. Heat the blueberries in a small pan over low heat for 5 minutes or until softened.
3. Add the water and potato starch to the blueberries.
4. Stir well and leave the berries to simmer for a further 2 minutes on low heat.
5. Meanwhile, melt the coconut oil with the palms of your hands.
6. Stir the oats, oat flour, melted coconut oil, salt, vanilla extract, and maple syrup together in a bowl until combined.
7. Pour the blueberries into a 9x13 baking dish and spread the crumble on top.
8. Bake the crumble for 30-35 minutes in the oven, or until the top has become crunchy and brown.

Per serving: Calories: 249 Protein: 3g Carbs: 35g Fiber: 4g Sugar: 15g Fat: 12g

Chocolate Quinoa Pudding Bars

SERVES 8 / PREP TIME: 10 MINUTES / COOK TIME: 25 MINUTES

A protein rich chocolate energy bar for a tempting dessert or snack.

---

1 small very ripe mashed banana
2 egg whites
¾ cup brown sugar
1 tsp vanilla extract
½ cup quinoa
¼ cup rice flour
1 tsp baking powder
1/4 cup cocoa powder, unsweetened

---

1. Preheat your oven to 350 degrees.
2. Line an 8-inch pan with parchment paper.
3. Mix the banana, egg whites, brown sugar and vanilla extract in a bowl.
4. Now mix in the quinoa, rice flour and baking powder.
5. Fold in the cocoa powder and then spread the batter out across the prepared pan.
6. Flatten the top with a cooking spatula or knife.
7. Bake for 25 minutes.
8. Allow the batter to cool before slicing into bars.

Per serving: Calories: 169 Protein: 3g Carbs: 39g Sugar: 24g Fat: 1g

50 SLOW COOKER
COOKBOOK RECIPES

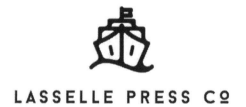

LASSELLE PRESS CO

BREAKFAST

One-Pot Breakfast

SERVES 4 / PREP TIME: 10 MINUTES / COOK TIME: 4 HOURS LOW

A delicious burst of energy to kick-start the day.

---

1 tbsp olive oil
2 white potatoes, peeled and sliced
1/2 red bell pepper diced
12 egg whites
1 cup almond milk
A pinch of salt and pepper

1 green onion stem, finely sliced (green section only)
8 oz crumbled goats cheese

---

1. Lightly rub the bottom of the slow cooker pan with oil.
2. Add half the potato slices followed by half the peppers.
3. Beat the egg whites and the milk together.
4. Season the liquid with a little salt and pepper to taste.
5. Add in the green onion and stir.
6. Pour the egg mixture into the pot over the potatoes.
7. Cook everything on Low for 4 hours.
8. In the last ten minutes, crumble on the goats cheese.
9. Enjoy a hearty breakfast.

Per serving: Calories: 366 Protein: 22g Carbs: 23g Fiber: 2g Sugar: 6g Fat: 20g (Unsaturated: 8g Saturated: 12g)

Sweet and Soft Raspberry Rice Pudding

SERVES 4 / PREP TIME: 10 MINUTES / COOK TIME: 1 HOUR HIGH

Sweet, juicy and warming. Perfect.

1/2 cup short grain rice
1 ½ tbsp chia seeds
2 cups water
3 cups almond milk
1/2 tsp ground cinnamon
Maple syrup to taste (optional)
2 cups organic raspberries

---

1. Combine the rice, chia seeds, water, almond milk, and cinnamon in the slow cooker. Mix well.
2. Cook on High for 1 hour.
3. Stir halfway through if you can.
4. Once the rice is thick and creamy, remove from the pot.
5. Place to one side and allow to cool for a few minutes.
6. Taste and stir in some maple syrup if desired.
7. Stir in the raspberries 15 minutes before serving.

Hint: If you have time, cook on Low for 4-5 hours instead for a really smooth, rich flavor.

Per serving: Calories: 216 Protein: 4g Carbs: 41g Fiber: 7g Sugar: 14g Fat: 4g (Unsaturated: 4g Saturated: 0g)

Sweetened Slow Oats

SERVES 3 / PREP TIME: 5 MINUTES / COOK TIME: 5 HOURS LOW

Just a great breakfast classic.

---

1 tsp coconut oil
1 cup steel-cut oats
2 cups almond milk
½ cup water
1/2 cup raisins
2 tbsp maple syrup
1 tbsp cinnamon

---

1. Rub the inside of your slow cooker with coconut oil.
2. Add all ingredients to the slow cooker – nice and simple.
3. Cook on Low for 5 hours.
4. Serve warm with a little dusting of extra cinnamon on top.

Hint: Soak your raisins for a few hours in warm water beforehand to plump them up. 8 tablespoons of raisins per serving are classed as low FODMAP.

Per serving: Calories: 273 Protein: 5g Carbs: 55g Fiber 6g: Sugar: 29g Fat: 5g (Unsaturated: 3g Saturated: 2g)

Fruity Quinoa Porridge

SERVES 4 / PREP TIME: 5 MINUTES / COOK TIME: 2 HOURS HIGH

Similar to oat porridge but with a slightly chunkier texture and higher in protein.

1 cup dry quinoa
3 cups almond milk
2 tsp cinnamon
1/4 tsp nutmeg
1 tsp vanilla extract
1 tsp brown sugar
1/4 tsp salt
2 medium bananas, sliced
1 cup organic blueberries

1. Throw all the ingredients (apart from the fresh fruit) into a slow cooker.
2. Cook on High for 2 hours or until all the liquid is absorbed.
3. Serve with the fresh fruit on top.

Hint: Alternatively, you can cook this on Low overnight for 7-8 hours to have it ready in the morning.

Per serving: Calories: 306 Protein: 7g Carbs: 60g Fiber: 7g Sugar: 24g Fat: 5g
(Unsaturated: 5g Saturated: 30)

Greek Red Pepper and Goats Cheese Frittata

SERVES 6 / PREP TIME: 10 MINUTES / COOK TIME:3 HOURS LOW

Bold Greek-inspired flavors; pair with a green salad!

1 tbsp olive oil
12 oz roasted red peppers, drained and cut into small pieces
½ cup pitted black olives, sliced
8 egg whites, beaten
1 tsp dried basil

4 oz crumbled goats cheese
1/4 cup sliced green onions (green tips only)
Fresh ground black pepper to taste

1. Rub the inside of the slow cooker with olive oil.
2. Add the red peppers and olives to the pot.
3. Whisk the egg whites with the basil and pour over the vegetables.
4. Using a fork, gently stir the mixture.
5. Sprinkle the crumbled cheese over the top.
6. Cook on Low for 3 hours or until the eggs are firm.
7. Cut into pieces while the frittata is still in the slow cooker.
8. Serve hot, sprinkled with chopped green onions.
9. Sprinkle with black pepper if desired.

Hint: As a rule of thumb, eggs are best when cooked as slowly as possible.

Per serving: Calories: 134 Protein: 8g Carbs: 6g Fiber: 1g Sugar: 3g Fat: 9g (Unsaturated: 5g Saturated: 4g)

Home Baked Pecan Loaf

SERVES 8 / PREP TIME: 10 MINUTES / COOK TIME: 1 HOUR

Not a slow cooker recipe but a staple you will probably want to have in your recipe bank!

Coconut oil as needed
1 1/2 cups rice flour
1/2 cup buckwheat flour
3 tsp baking powder
1/2 tsp salt

2 tbsp coconut sugar
2 egg whites
1 cup unsweetened almond milk
1/2 cup coconut oil
2 tbsp crushed pecan nuts

---

1. Preheat the oven to 350 degrees.
2. Grease a loaf pan generously with coconut oil.
3. Sift together the rice flour, the buckwheat flour, the baking powder, and the salt into a large bowl.
4. Stir in the sugar.
5. Meanwhile, using an electric mixer, lightly beat the egg whites until they are just frothy.
6. Stir in the milk and the coconut oil.
7. Now pour the flour mixture into the bowl with the egg white mixture.
8. Beat on a medium speed for 2 to 3 minutes, or until smooth.
9. Pour this mixture into the greased loaf pan.
10. Smooth the top with a spatula.
11. Next, sprinkle the crushed pecans over the top of the mixture, pressing them down slightly.
12. Bake for 55 minutes to 1 hour, testing to see if a toothpick or knife comes out clean.
13. Set the pan to cool on a wire rack for at least 10 minutes.
14. Turn the bread out onto the wire rack to finish cooling.

Hint: You can substitute other gluten free flours in place of the rice and buckwheat flours depending on what you have in your cupboards!

Per serving: Calories: 268   Protein: 6g Carbs: 37g Sugar: 3g Fat: 18g

POULTRY

Rich Coq au Vin Stew

SERVES 6 / PREP TIME: 10 MINUTES / COOK TIME: 6 HOURS LOW

A classic French-inspired stew with warming flavors.

Olive oil cooking spray
16 oz chicken breasts, skinless and boneless
1 cup red wine
2 cups water
1 cup diced carrot
½ cup sliced green onion, (green tips only)
2 tbsp dried oregano
2 whole bay leaves
½ tsp dried thyme
½ cup low FODMAP chicken stock
2 tbsp tomato paste

---

1. Spray a large skillet with cooking oil, over medium heat.
2. Add the chicken and brown it evenly, turning occasionally.
3. Remove the chicken and add to the bottom of your slow cooker.
4. Use 1/2 of the red wine to de-glaze the skillet.
5. (Hint: Make sure to scrape up all the brown bits – that's the good stuff.)
6. Pour the wine from the skillet into the slow cooker.
7. Add the remaining wine, water, vegetables, herbs, stock and paste.
8. Stir to evenly distribute the ingredients in the slow cooker.
9. Cover and cook on Low 6 hours until the chicken and vegetables are tender.
10. Remove bay leaves before serving.

Per serving: Calories: 178 Protein: 24g Carbs: 6g Fiber: 2g Sugar: 2g Fat: 3g (Unsaturated: 2g Saturated: 1g)

Wild Rice and Chicken Stock

SERVES 4 / PREP TIME: 5 MINUTES / COOK TIME: 4 HOURS + 30 MINUTES HIGH

A slow cooking winter warming stock with an added flair.

---

4 carrots, peeled and chopped
1 large zucchini, chopped
16oz boneless, skinless chicken breasts, halved
1 tbsp unsalted butter
1/2 tsp dried oregano
1 bay leaf
4 cups low FODMAP chicken stock
1 cup water

3/4 cup wild rice
1 tsp garlic-infused olive oil
1 green onion, (green tips only), sliced
3 tbsp lemon juice
A pinch of salt and black pepper to taste
1 tbsp chopped fresh Italian parsley for serving

---

1. Add the first 8 ingredients to a large slow cooker.
2. Cook until the chicken is cooked through and the rice is tender (4 hours on High).
3. Transfer the chicken breasts to a cutting board and allow to cool slightly.
4. Meanwhile, heat the butter in a skillet on medium heat.
5. Add the onion and sauté until tender for 6 to 8 minutes.
6. Shred the chicken with a knife and fork and add it back to the slow cooker with the onion.
7. Cover and cook until the chicken is heated through (30 minutes on High).
8. Add water or stock to thin to your desired consistency.
9. Turn off the slow cooker and stir in the lemon juice.
10. Season to taste with salt and black pepper.
11. Ladle into bowls and top with fresh parsley.

Per serving: Calories: 254 Protein:28g Carbs: 17g Fiber: 2g Sugar: 4g Fat: 8g (Unsaturated: 6g Saturated: 2g)

Tender Turkey Wraps

SERVES 8 / PREP TIME: 10 MINUTES / COOK TIME: 7 HOURS LOW

Nice and healthy and packed with flavor.

---

1 lb turkey breasts, skinless and boneless
14.5 oz can low sodium diced tomatoes
1 cup water
1 tbsp dried parsley
3/4 tbsp sea salt
1/4 tbsp black pepper
8 6" rice/corn tortillas
2 cups pineapple chunks (or 1 can Dole sliced pineapple)

1 cup raw spinach, washed
1/4 cup fresh cilantro, chopped

Lime dressing:

1/4 cup lime juice
1/4 cup olive oil
1/2 tsp sugar
1/4 tsp salt

---

1. Spray the bottom of your slow cooker with cooking spray.
2. Place the turkey breasts in the cooker.
3. Add in the tomatoes, water, parsley, salt and pepper. Stir to combine.
4. Cover and cook on Low for 7 hours.
5. Prepare the lime dressing by mixing all the ingredients, cover and chill in the refrigerator.
6. After 7 hours, carefully remove the turkey with meat claws and shred (alternatively use two forks) and place to one side.
7. With a spoon, top each tortilla with 1/8 cup the turkey meat.
8. Divide the pineapple among the tortillas.
9. Toss the spinach and the cilantro with the lime dressing.
10. Top the tortillas with the salad and wrap into neat parcels.

Hint: There will be a nice thick sauce in the bottom of the slow cooker - use in the wraps if desired.

Per serving: Calories: 199 Protein: 14g Carbs: 19g Fiber: 3g Sugar: 6g Fat: 8g (Unsaturated: 7g Saturated: 1g)

Slow Cooker Turkey Masala Curry

SERVES 4 / PREP TIME: 10 MINUTES / COOK TIME: 1 HOUR 45 MINUTES LOW

Soft, juicy and delicately spiced.

---

1 lb skinless and boneless turkey
breasts, cut into 2" slices
1 (14.5 oz) can diced tomatoes
1 tsp curry powder
1 tsp garam masala
1 tsp salt
1/2 tsp Asafoetida Powder
1/4 tsp dried cilantro

1/2 cup dairy-free sour cream/yogurt
(optional)

---

1. Add all the ingredients (except the sour cream) into a food processor.
2. Grind until fully blended.
3. Add your spice mixture to the slow cooker.
4. Add your turkey slices. Cover.
5. Cook on Low for 1 hour 45 minutes until turkey is thoroughly cooked through.
6. Add the sour cream/yoghurt and swirl through.
7. Serve with rice if desired.

Per serving: Calories: 185 Protein: 25g Carbs: 7g Fiber: 1g Sugar: 0g Fat: 6g
(Unsaturated: 0g Saturated: 5g)

Turkey-Stuffed Red Peppers

SERVES 6 / PREP TIME: 15 MINUTES / COOK TIME: 7-8 HOURS LOW

Tasty, herby and rich with melting cheese.

---

1 lb lean ground turkey
1 cup uncooked white rice
8 oz goats cheese, crumbled
1 tbsp diced chives
1 tsp salt
1/2 tsp ground black pepper
1 tsp dried rosemary
6 large red bell peppers, tops cut off
and de-seeded

Sauce:

32 oz fresh beef tomatoes, diced and
juices reserved
2 tsp minced fresh parsley
1 tsp dried oregano
1 tsp brown sugar
A pinch of baking soda
1 ½ cups low FODMAP vegetable stock

---

1. Mix together the first 7 ingredients for the stuffing.
2. Stuff evenly into the peppers, about 3/4 of the way full.
3. Spray the inside of your slow cooker with cooking oil.
4. Place the stuffed peppers inside.
5. Combine the first 5 ingredients of the sauce.
6. Pour this sauce over the peppers, then pour the stock around the sides into the base of the slow cooker pan.
7. Cover and cook on Low for 7 to 8 hours.

Per serving: Calories: 382 Protein: 25g Carbs: 26g Fiber: 2g Sugar: 7g Fat: 20g
(Unsaturated: 9g Saturated: 10g)

Hearty Turkey and Vegetable Casserole

SERVES 4 / PREP TIME: 10 MINUTES / COOK TIME: 8 HOURS LOW

Wonderfully warming with chunky vegetables.

1½ cups leek (green tips only)
3 cups parsnip, peeled and cubed
2 large carrots
10 oz potatoes, peeled and cubed
12 oz lean turkey breasts, skinless and boneless
1 tbsp olive oil
1 tsp dried oregano

1/2 tsp dried thyme
4 cups low FODMAP chicken stock
1 cup boiling water
1 tbsp ground black pepper
6oz green beans
3 tbsp fresh parsley

---

1. Spray the bottom of your slow cooker dish with cooking oil.
2. Turn the cooker onto the Low setting.
3. Roughly chop the leeks, parsnips, carrots and potatoes into cubes.
4. Add the turkey to the slow cooker.
5. Add the vegetables.
6. Add the olive oil, dried oregano and thyme.
7. Pour the stock into the slow cooker.
8. Add the boiling water along with the black pepper.
9. Leave the slow cooker to cook on Low for 8 hours.
10. Check the stew after this time – if a little bit dry, add some boiling water until the ingredients are just covered.
11. Trim the green beans.
12. Blanch in a small saucepan for 2 to 3 minutes until tender.
13. Stir them through the stew.
14. Divide the stew into bowls and garnish with fresh parsley. Enjoy!

Per serving: Calories: 387 Protein: 27g Carbs: 52g Fiber: 10g Sugar: 10g Fat: 9g (Unsaturated: 7g Saturated: 2g)

Chicken Meatballs with Fluffy Rice

SERVES 8 / PREP TIME: 10 MINUTES / COOK TIME: 3 HOURS LOW/1.5 HOURS HIGH

Tender, juicy meatballs in a tangy tomato sauce.

---

1 celery stick, sliced
2 small carrots, peeled and sliced
4 5oz skinless chicken breasts, sliced
2 tbsp chives (green tips only)
1 tbsp olive oil, for greasing
1 cup tomato paste
1 cup low FODMAP chicken stock

1 cup beef tomatoes, sliced
2 cups cooked white rice

---

1. Blend the celery, carrots, chicken and chives in a food processor.
2. Shape into small meatballs with the palms of your hands.
3. To cook, grease the slow cooker with olive oil.
4. Add the meatballs, tomato paste and chicken stock to combine.
5. Cook on High for 3 hours on Low or 1 1/2 hours on High.
6. Add the fresh tomatoes 15 minutes before serving.
7. Served with freshly cooked rice.

Tip: This is a high protein dish so please keep track of your daily protein intake compared to the average recommendations – this will make up 50% of this amount! Great if you're working out, or not getting much protein from your other meals.

Per serving: Calories: 220 Protein: 24.5g Carbs: 20g Fiber: 2.5g Sugar:5.5g Fat: 5g (Unsaturated: 4g Saturated: 1g)

Italian-Seasoned Chicken Bake

SERVES 8 / PREP TIME: 15 MINUTES / COOK TIME: 5 HOURS LOW

Very easy and delicious, sure to be a weekly favorite.

---

1 tbsp olive oil
4 5oz skinless chicken breasts
1 stick of celery, finely chopped
1 carrot, peeled and finely diced
14 oz fresh beef tomatoes, quartered
1 cup low FODMAP chicken stock
1 tbsp tomato paste

1 tbsp garlic-infused oil
1 tsp brown sugar
1 tbsp fresh basil, torn
A pinch of salt and pepper
1lb 5oz potatoes, peeled and cubed
1 tbsp chopped fresh chives (green tips only) to garnish

---

1. Heat a large saucepan over medium heat.
2. Add the oil and, once hot, add the chicken breasts.
3. Brown the chicken for about 3-4 minutes, or until golden-brown.
4. Remove from the pan and add to the slow cooker.
5. Add the celery and carrot and stir.
6. Pour over the tomatoes, stock, paste, garlic oil, sugar and basil.
7. Mix well to make sure everything is evenly distributed.
8. Season with a little salt and pepper if desired.
9. Cover with a lid and cook on Low for 5 hours.
10. Add the potatoes with one hour to go.
11. Serve with a scatter of chives.

Hint: As this meal serves 8, portion up the leftovers and freeze in an airtight container for 2-3 weeks.

Per serving: Calories: 200 Protein: 18.5g Carbs: 18g Fiber: 3g Sugar: 3g Fat: 5.5g (Unsaturated: 4.5g Saturated: 1g)

Chicken and Olive Bake

SERVES 5 /   PREP TIME: 10 MINUTES /   COOK TIME: 5 HOURS HIGH/ 8 HOURS LOW

The tender chicken pairs really well with the saltiness of the olives.

---

1 tbsp olive oil
12oz skinless chicken breasts
2 slices of preserved lemon
½ cup pitted black olives, whole
2 tsp dried cilantro
2 tsp cumin
1 cup low FODMAP vegetable stock
1 tbsp low sodium tomato paste

---

1. Brown the chicken over medium-high heat in a little olive oil.
2. Add the chicken to the slow cooker.
3. Add in the rest of the ingredients and stir together well.
4. Cover and cook on High for 5 hours or Low for 8 hours.
5. Serve alongside your choice of rice or quinoa.

Hint: If you're watching your sodium intake you can rinse the olives before cooking.)

Hint: As this meal serves 8, portion up the leftovers and freeze in an airtight container for 2-3 weeks.

Per serving: Calories: 157 Protein: 21g Carbs: 2g Fiber: 1g Sugar: 1g Fat: 7g (Unsaturated: 6g Saturated: 1g)

Tunisian Chicken

SERVES 8 / PREP TIME: 10 MINUTES / COOK TIME: 5 HOURS HIGH/ 8 HOURS LOW

Nicely spiced and full of flavor.

4x 5oz chicken breast fillets
2 white potatoes, peeled and cut into 1in cubes
2 carrots, peeled and cut into 1in cubes
1 tbsp olive oil
1 stalk of celery, sliced
1 tsp cumin
1 tsp turmeric
1 tbsp fresh cilantro

1 lemon, quartered
1 cup beef tomatoes, quartered

---

1. Brown the chicken over medium-high heat in a little olive oil.
2. Keep the lemon and tomatoes to one side for now.
3. Into the slow cooker, add the chicken with the rest of the ingredients and stir well.
4. Cover and cook on High for 5 hours or Low for 8 hours.
5. Add the tomatoes for the last hour.
6. Serve alongside rice with a wedge of lemon.
7. Finish by garnishing with a scattering of fresh cilantro.

Hint: As this meal serves 8, portion up the leftovers and freeze in an airtight container for 2-3 weeks.

Per serving: Calories: 150 Protein: 17g Carbs: 11.5g Fiber: 2g Sugar: 1.5g Fat: 4g (Unsaturated: 3g Saturated: 1g)

Tangy Orange Chicken

SERVES 8 / PREP TIME: 15 MINUTES / COOK TIME: 4 HOURS HIGH/7 HOURS LOW

A classic combination of citrus and juicy chicken.

2 tbsp olive oil
4 5oz boneless skinless chicken
breasts
2 cup water
1 fresh orange, sliced
1 tsp dried cilantro
2 cups low FODMAP chicken stock
4 slices of preserved lemon
½ cup fresh parsley, chopped

1. Heat the oil in a skillet over medium heat.
2. Season the chicken and add to the pan.
3. Sauté for 4 minutes each side until browned all over.
4. Remove and set aside.
5. Into the slow cooker add the water, orange slices, cilantro and stock.
6. Stir in the chicken and preserved lemon.
7. Cook on Low for 7-8 hours or High for 4-5 hours.
8. Finish by garnishing with a little bit of parsley.

Hint: As this meal serves 8, portion up the leftovers and freeze in an airtight container for 2-3 weeks.

Per serving: Calories: 135 Protein: 17.5g Carbs: 3g Fiber: 0.5g Sugar: 1.5g Fat: 5.5g (Unsaturated: 4.5g Saturated: 1g)

SOUPS AND STOCKS

Slow Cooker Chicken Soup

SERVES 4 / PREP TIME: 10 MINUTES / COOK TIME: 6 HOURS LOW

This classic dish tastes wonderful after cooking all day—and smells good too!

Olive oil cooking spray
1 lb skinless chicken breasts
2 large carrots, peeled and chopped
2 parsnips, peeled and chopped
1/2 cup chives (green tips only), finely chopped
2 tbsp garlic-infused oil
1 tbsp fresh lemon juice
1/2 tsp dried thyme
1/2 tsp dried rosemary

1/2 tsp dried oregano
2 dried bay leaves
4 cups low FODMAP chicken stock
A pinch of salt to taste
3 tbsp fresh parsley, finely chopped
1 tbsp fresh cilantro, chopped

---

1. Spray the slow cooker dish with cooking spray.
2. Line the bottom of the slow cooker with the chicken breasts.
3. Cover with the carrots, parsnips, chives, garlic-infused oil, fresh lemon juice, thyme, rosemary, oregano, and bay leaves.
4. Cover everything with the low FODMAP chicken stock.
5. Season with a pinch of salt to taste.
6. Place the lid on the slow cooker.
7. Cook on Low for 6 hours.
8. Just before serving, remove chicken, allow to cool and shred using two forks.
9. Return to the soup and stir well.
10. Dish the hot chicken soup into bowls and sprinkle with the parsley and cilantro to serve.

Per serving: Calories: 276 Protein: 32g Carbs: 20g Fiber: 4g Sugar: 6g Fat: 8g

Warming Potato Soup

SERVES 8 / PREP TIME: 10 MINUTES / COOK TIME: 6-7 HOURS LOW

Perfect for cold days to warm you up.

---

5 medium baking potatoes, peeled and cubed (4-5 cups)
2 large carrots, thinly sliced in rounds
1 tbsp olive oil
1 tbsp butter
1/2 tsp salt
1/2 tsp ground black pepper

2 cups low FODMAP chicken stock
1/2 cup cottage cheese
2 tbsp cornstarch/potato starch

---

1. Place first 7 ingredients in the slow cooker, stirring well.
2. Cover and cook on Low for 6-7 hours.
3. When ready to serve, add the cheese.
4. Stir until lumps dissolve.
5. To thicken the soup, add the starch and stir well.

Hint: If you prefer a thinner soup, leave the starch out.

Per serving: Calories: 193 Protein: 5g Carbs: 26g Fiber: 3g Sugar: 2g Fat: 8g (Unsaturated: 2g Saturated: 5g)

Wholesome Tomato Pasta Soup

SERVES 5 / PREP TIME: 5 MINUTES / COOK TIME: 4 HOURS HIGH/8 HOURS LOW

An old-time favorite with a little something extra.

---

28 oz canned tomatoes
1 tsp olive oil
2 tbsp brown sugar
1 tsp dried oregano
1 tsp dried rosemary
1 tsp sea salt
1/2 tsp ground black pepper
6 cups low FODMAP chicken stock

1/2 cup tomato paste
3 cups cooked gluten free elbow macaroni

---

1. Add the tomatoes, oil, sugar, herbs, salt, pepper, and stock to your slow cooker pan.
2. Cook on High for 4 hours or Low for 8 hours.
3. 20 minutes before serving, mix in the tomato paste and the pasta.
4. Serve steaming hot in nice big bowls.

Per serving: Calories: 230 Protein:13g Carbs:40g Fiber: 9g Sugar: 15g Fat: 4g (Unsaturated: 3g Saturated: 1g)

Classic Creamy Tomato Soup

SERVES 5 / PREP TIME: 5 MINUTES / COOK TIME: 4 HOURS HIGH/8 HOURS LOW

Hot and delicious, perfect for a hot lunch or as a starter.

---

28 oz can of crushed tomatoes
4 cups low FODMAP chicken stock
1 tsp oregano
1 tbsp garlic-infused oil
1 tsp brown sugar
1 tsp ground black pepper
1 cup dairy free cream or rice milk

---

1. Add tomatoes, chicken stock, oregano and oil to the crock pot.
2. Add in the sugar and pepper.
3. Stir well.
4. Cook on High for 4 hours or Low for 8 hours.
5. Strain the soup and purée any chunks in a blender.
6. (Hint: You can also blend with an immersion blender for a very smooth consistency.)
7. Return the soup to the slow cooker.
8. Add cream/milk and stir well.

Per serving: Calories: 181 Protein: 6g Carbs: 12g Fiber: 3g Sugar: 8g Fat: 13g (Unsaturated: 4g Saturated: 9g)

Rustic Fish Stock

SERVES 8 / PREP TIME: 20 MINUTES / COOK TIME: 1 HOUR ON LOW

This works as a great base for noodle dishes, sauces or fish soups.

3 lb fish bones, including heads
10 cups water
3 green onion stalks, (green tips only)
chopped
2 zucchinis, roughly sliced

1. Place the fish bones and water to a large pan and bring to the boil over high heat.
2. Lower to medium and simmer for 20 minutes, then pass through a strainer into the slow cooker.
3. Add the vegetables to the slow cooker and cook on Low for 1 hour.
4. Strain again, then use straight away or store.

Hint: You can store stock in a sealable container in the fridge for up to 4 days. Otherwise, store it in portions in the freezer for 2-3 weeks.

Per serving: Calories: 65 Protein: 11g Carbs: 4g Fiber: 1g Sugar: 2g Fat: 1g (Unsaturated: 0g Saturated: 0g)

Low FODMAP Chicken Stock

SERVES 6 / PREP TIME: 10 MINUTES / COOK TIME: 6 HOURS ON LOW

Incredibly versatile, a great base for many recipes in this cookbook.

2-3 lb whole chicken (thighs, breasts and legs cut up)
2 celery stalks with leaves, diced
2 medium carrots, chopped
2 tsp dried thyme
2 green onion stalks, (green tips only) chopped

½ tsp dried oregano
10 whole black peppercorns
5-7 cups cold water (to fully cover ingredients)

---

1. Place all the ingredients in a large slow cooker.
2. Cover and cook on Low for 6 hours.
3. Gently remove the chicken from the stock and set aside.
4. Strain the stock and discard the vegetables.
5. (Hint: Alternatively, keep the vegetables and use them for a soup.)
6. Use immediately or store for later.
7. Once cooled, you can skim the fat from the surface to use.

Hint: You can store stock in a sealable container in the fridge for up to 4 days. Otherwise, store it in portions in the freezer for 2-3 weeks.

Per serving: Calories: 188 Protein: 24g Carbs: 4g Fiber: 1g Sugar: 1g Fat: 8g (Unsaturated: 5g Saturated: 2g)

Low FODMAP Vegetable Stock

SERVES 6 / PREP TIME: 5 MINUTES / COOK TIME: 6 HOURS ON LOW

A great veggie alternative for soups, sauces or as a base for many recipes.

---

2 celery stalks, roughly chopped
2 large carrots, roughly chopped
1 cup rutabaga, peeled and chopped
3 bay leaves
2 tsp dried oregano
2 sprigs of fresh rosemary
2 sprigs of fresh thyme
1 bunch fresh chives, chopped (green tips only)
5 whole black peppercorns

A pinch of salt
5-7 cups cold water (to fully cover ingredients)

---

1. Place all the ingredients into a large slow cooker.
2. Cover and cook on Low for 6 hours.
3. Skim the foam that may have risen to the top.
4. Pass the stock through a fine sieve.
5. Discard vegetables and herbs.
6. Allow to cool.

Hint: You can store stock in a sealable container in the fridge for up to 4 days. Otherwise, store it in portions in the freezer for 2-3 weeks.

Per serving: Calories: 26 Protein: 1g Carbs: 6g Fiber: 2g Sugar: 3g Fat:0g (Unsaturated: 0g Saturated: 0g)

VEGETARIAN

Indulgent Macaroni and Goats Cheese

SERVES 8 / PREP TIME: 10 MINUTES / COOK TIME: 3 HOURS LOW

A perfect bowl of comfort food; it's okay to treat yourself once in a while!

Olive oil cooking spray
1 egg white
½ lb dry gluten free macaroni (approx. 1/2 box)
2 ½ cups goat milk
2 tbsp unsalted butter, diced
2 cups goats cheese, crumbled

---

1. Spray the base and sides of your slow cooker with olive oil cooking spray.
2. (Hint: This keeps the macaroni from sticking to the sides of the cooker.)
3. Pour the beaten egg white into the slow cooker.
4. Add the dry macaroni.
5. Pour in the milk.
6. Add the butter.
7. Sprinkle in a little salt (if desired).
8. Crumble the cheese into the pot.
9. Stir the ingredients well to mix.
10. Cook on Low for 3 hours.

Per serving: Calories: 262 Protein: 14g Carbs: 25g Fiber: 1g Sugar: 2g Fat: 11g (Unsaturated: 7g Saturated: 8g)

Easy Jacket Potatoes

SERVES 6 / PREP TIME: 10 MINUTES / COOK TIME: 4 HOURS HIGH/8 HOURS LOW

A great lunch or side with your favorite topping.

---

6 large baking potatoes
1 ½ tbsp coconut oil
A pinch of celery salt to taste
Fresh ground pepper to taste
Your choice of low FODMAP topping

---

1. Scrub and dry the potatoes.
2. Pierce each potato a few times with a fork.
3. Rub each potato with a little coconut oil (use paper towel or your fingers).
4. Season with celery salt, and pepper and wrap in aluminum foil.
5. Place in the slow cooker.
6. Cook on High for 4 hours or Low for 8 hours.
7. Enjoy with a knob of butter or your choice of topping – goats cheese and tomatoes work well or you could try cottage cheese and chopped green chives with a squeeze of lemon.

(Without topping:)
Per serving: Calories: 246 Protein: 6g Carbs: 49g Fiber: 6g Sugar: 2g Fat: 4g
(Unsaturated: 0g Saturated: 3g)

Bubbling Tomato and Pepper Pasta Bake

SERVES 6 / PREP TIME: 10 MINUTES / COOK TIME: 3 HOURS LOW

A great plate of soft pasta in a rich Italian sauce.

---

4 cups gluten free pasta shapes of your choice
2 red bell peppers, diced
2 green bell peppers, diced
1 cup low FODMAP vegetable stock
2 cups beef tomatoes, diced

A pinch of salt and pepper
1 tsp dried oregano
1 tsp dried rosemary
3 cups fresh spinach

---

1. Add the pasta and peppers to the slow cooker and mix well.
2. Pour in the stock and beef tomatoes and stir to combine.
3. Sprinkle in the salt and pepper, then add the herbs.
4. Cook on High for 3 hours.
5. Add the spinach about 30 minutes before serving until wilted.
6. Spoon onto plates and enjoy.

Per serving: Calories: 312 Protein: 12g Carbs: 62g Fiber: 6g Sugar: 6g Fat: 2g (Unsaturated: 1g Saturated: 0g)

Root Vegetables, Quinoa and Herbs

SERVES 2 / PREP TIME: 5 MINUTES / COOK TIME: 5 HOURS LOW/1 HOUR HIGH

Winter vegetables with soft, tasty quinoa.

1 cup quinoa
1 cup beef tomatoes, coarsely chopped
1 tbsp dried oregano
1 tsp dried thyme
2 medium carrots, diced
½ rutabaga, peeled and diced
1 cup pumpkin, diced

A pinch of salt
1 cup water
1 cup fresh spinach

1. Add all the ingredients to the slow cooker and stir well.
2. Cook everything on Low for 5 hours or High for 1 hour, or until the quinoa has soaked up most of the liquid.
3. Serve and enjoy.

Hint: To speed up the cooking process you can soak the quinoa overnight in double the amount of water as quinoa. Reduce cooking time by half and leave out the water when cooking.

Per serving: Calories: 427 Protein: 16g Carbs: 82g Fiber: 16g Sugar: 16g Fat: 6g (Unsaturated: 4g Saturated: 1g)

Potato Dauphinoise

SERVES 5 / PREP TIME: 5 MINUTES / COOK TIME: 1-2 HOURS HIGH

Wonderfully creamy and perfect as a side or a casserole topping.

---

5 medium white potatoes, peeled and
thinly sliced
1 tbsp olive oil
2 tbsp potato starch
1 cup rice milk
1½ tsp salt
1 tsp dried parsley
A pinch of black pepper
1 tbsp fresh thyme

---

1. Start by layering the potatoes in the bottom of the slow cooker.
2. Make sure it's 3 layers deep and the base is fully covered.
3. For the béchamel, use a medium saucepan to heat the olive oil over medium-low heat until melted.
4. Add the potato starch and stir until smooth.
5. Cook until the mixture turns light golden, about 5 minutes.
6. Slowly add the milk to the mixture, whisking continuously until smooth.
7. Bring to a rolling boil over high heat.
8. Cook for 10 minutes over medium heat, stirring constantly, then remove from heat.
9. Season with salt, parsley and pepper.
10. Pour this over the potatoes in the slow cooker.
11. Cook on High for 1-2 hours until bubbling.
12. Finish with a scattering of fresh thyme.

Per serving: Calories: 153 Protein: 5g Carbs: 35g Fiber: 2g Sugar: 5g Fat: 1g
(Unsaturated: 1g Saturated: 0g)

Winter Stew with Parsnip and Fennel

SERVES 5 / PREP TIME: 5 MINUTES / COOK TIME: 4 HOURS LOW

Delicious and brilliantly simple.

---

2 cups low FODMAP vegetable stock
2 cups parsnip, peeled and cubed
3 or 4 collard green leaves, ribs removed + chopped
5 small fennel hearts
1 tbsp garlic-infused oil
3 bay leaves
1 tsp turmeric

1 tsp dried parsley
A pinch of ground celery seed
A pinch of dried rosemary
A pinch of salt to taste
A pinch of coarse ground pepper, to taste

---

1. Combine all the ingredients and cook on Low for 4 hours (or until all the veggies are tender.)
2. Remove the bay leaves before spooning into bowls.

Per serving: Calories: 129 Protein: 5g Carbs: 23g Fiber: 7g Sugar: 9g Fat: 4g (Unsaturated: 3g Saturated: 1g)

Vegan Sweet and Sour

SERVES 5 / PREP TIME: 5 MINUTES / COOK TIME: 7 HOURS LOW

Delicious bold flavors, serve with rice or as a sauce for noodles.

---

2 ½ cups low FODMAP vegetable stock
2 cups water
1 tbsp tomato paste
2 tbsp extra virgin olive oil
4 stalks of celery, chopped
1 bok choy plant
1/2 cup carrots chopped
1 zucchini, diced
½ cup pineapple
A pinch of salt and pepper

---

1. Heat the stock and water in a pan over high heat - bring to a boil.
2. Stir through the tomato paste.
3. Add the rest of the ingredients to the slow cooker.
4. Pour the liquid over the vegetables.
5. Cook on Low for 7 hours.

Per serving: Calories: 97 Protein: 3g Carbs: 10g Fiber: 3g Sugar: 6g Fat: 6g
(Unsaturated: 5g Saturated: 1g)

Quinoa and Slow Roasted Red Peppers

SERVES 8 / PREP TIME: 15 MINUTES / COOK TIME: LOW 8 HOURS/ HIGH 3 - 4 HOURS

Roasted peppers add a sweet, smoky taste to the quinoa.

2 medium red peppers
1 medium green pepper, diced (about 1½ cup)
4 cups low FODMAP vegetable stock
1 tsp dried oregano
2 tsp ground cumin
¼ tsp thyme
1 tsp sea salt

¾ cup uncooked quinoa, rinsed under cold water and drained
4 cup green beans, ends trimmed
8 lemon wedges
2 tbsp fresh cilantro, chopped

1. First, roast your peppers: turn the oven on to the highest broil setting.
2. Move the rack to about 1/3 of the way from the top of the oven.
3. Wash and dry the whole peppers and place them on a baking sheet.
4. Place in the oven and broil for 2-3 minute.
5. Make sure the tops are slightly blackened.
6. Turn them with tongs and continue broiling until most sides are blistered and blackened.
7. Remove the peppers from the oven.
8. Make a tent with a large piece of foil over the top of the peppers to let them sweat.
9. Meanwhile, add stock, oregano, cumin, thyme, and salt to the slow cooker.
10. Add quinoa and stir.
11. Carefully peel the skin off of the peppers.
12. Remove the stem and the seeds, too.
13. Dice and add to the slow cooker.
14. Stir gently to mix all of the ingredients together.
15. Cook on Low for 8 hours or on High for 3 - 4 hours or until the quinoa is tender.
16. Add in the green beans 30 minutes before the end.
17. Scoop into bowls and squeeze a lemon wedge over each serving before garnishing with cilantro to finish.

Per serving: Calories: 119 Protein: 5g Carbs: 20g Fiber: 4g Sugar: 4g Fat: 3g (Unsaturated: 1g Saturated: 2g)

Greek Olive and Pepper Rice

SERVES 8 / PREP TIME: 10 MINUTES / COOK TIME: 1 1/2 HOURS + 30 MINUTES HIGH

Soft, sweet peppers, salty olives and tasty rice.

2 tbsp garlic-infused olive oil
2 cups white rice
3 cups low FODMAP vegetable stock
4 cups water
1 red bell pepper, seeds removed and finely chopped
1 green bell pepper, seeds removed and finely chopped
1 tsp dried rosemary

1 ½ cups goats cheese
3/4 cup sliced black olives, pitted
2 tbsp fresh-squeezed lemon juice
A pinch of salt and fresh-ground black pepper to taste
1/4 cup sliced green onions (green tips only)

1. Heat the olive oil in a large heavy frying pan over medium heat.
2. Add the rice and sauté for 5 minutes, or until the rice is nicely browned.
3. Put the browned rice into the slow cooker.
4. Add the stock and water to the pan to remove any browned bits.
5. Add the de-glazed mixture to the cooker with the rice.
6. Cook on High for 1 ½ hours.
7. After 1 ½ hours add the peppers and cook for 15 minutes more.
8. Add in the rosemary at this point.
9. Add 1 cup of the cheese and all of the sliced olives to the slow cooker.
10. Cook for another 15 minutes.
11. Check the rice is cooked through, then stir in the lemon juice.
12. Season with salt and fresh-ground pepper to taste.
13. Top with additional crumbled goats cheese and green onions as desired.
14. Serve it hot.

Per serving: Calories: 306 Protein: 11g Carbs: 37g Fiber: 1g Sugar: 2g Fat: 13g
(Unsaturated: 6g Saturated: 6g)

SEAFOOD

Tomato and Olive Fish Stew

SERVING SIZE: 4 / PREP TIME: 10 MINUTES / COOK TIME: 7-8 HOURS LOW /3-4 HOURS HIGH

Delicate fish with the tang of capers and tomatoes.

4x 5oz white fish fillets
½ tsp capers
3 medium potatoes, sliced into 1cm/ half-inch thick slices
2 cups beef tomatoes, chopped
1 cup water

1 cup dry white wine
3 tbsp fresh parsley, chopped
½ cup pitted black olives
A pinch of sea salt
A pinch of oregano

1. Combine all ingredients in a slow cooker and cook on Low for 7-8 hours or High for 3-4 hours until fish is flaky.
2. Flake the fish fillets with a knife and fork and stir well.
3. Serve up with your choice of rice or potatoes.

Per serving: Calories: 304 Protein: 28g Carbs: 31g Fiber: 4g Sugar: 4g Fat: 3g (Unsaturated: 2g Saturated: 0g)

Spiced Fish Stew

SERVES: 6 / PREP TIME: 10 MINUTES / COOK TIME: LOW 7-8 HOURS/HIGH 3-4 HOURS

Cod absorbs the delicious flavors it is cooked in.

2 tsp ground ginger
1 tsp ground cumin
1 tsp turmeric
1 lemon, juiced
2 cups fresh beef tomatoes, diced
1 tbsp chopped chives
1lb 2oz firm cod fillets
A pinch of salt and freshly ground
black pepper

1. Combine all ingredients in a slow cooker.
2. Cook on Low for 7-8 hours or High for 3-4 hours until fish is flaky.
3. Flake the cod fillets with a knife and fork and stir gently.
4. Serve with rice.

Hint: Season the fish with lemon, salt and pepper before cooking and leave to marinate over night if you have time.

Per serving: Calories: 79 Protein: 14g Carbs: 4g Fiber: 1g Sugar: 2g Fat: 1g (Unsaturated: 0g Saturated: 0g)

Spiced Shrimp Curry

SERVES 4 / PREP TIME: 10 MINUTES / COOK TIME: 1 HOUR + 15 MINUTES LOW

Succulently spiced, meaty shrimp in a tomato and ginger based curry.

---

1 tsp cumin seeds
1 tsp coriander seeds
1 tsp fenugreek seeds
2 cups chopped tomatoes
1 thumb-sized piece of fresh ginger
1 tsp garlic-infused oil
1 tsp dried dill

1 cup low FODMAP vegetable stock
1 tbsp maple syrup
10½ oz shrimp, heads and shells removed, de-veined
1 tbsp lemon juice

---

1. For the curry sauce, heat a frying pan over medium heat.
2. Add the spices and dry fry for 2-3 minutes, or until fragrant.
3. Transfer the spices to a mortar and pestle and grind to a powder.
4. Add the tomatoes, ginger, garlic oil and dill to the slow cooker.
5. Add the stock and maple syrup and cook on Low for 1 hour.
6. Add the shrimp to the slow cooker and cook for a further 15-20 minutes on high or until shrimp is cooked through.
7. Serve with your choice of rice and a squeeze of fresh lemon.

Per serving: Calories: 139 Protein: 19g Carbs: 9g Fiber: 1g Sugar: 6g Fat: 3g
(Unsaturated: 3g Saturated: 0g)

Fresh Spanish-Inspired Mussels

SERVES 6 / PREP TIME: 10 MINUTES / COOK TIME: 2 HOURS + 10 MINUTES LOW

Deliciously tender mussels with a rich sauce.

---

1 red pepper, de-seeded and sliced
2 cups paella rice
1 cup chopped tomatoes
2 cups low FODMAP fish stock, heated through

1 cup fresh mussels (meat or in shell)
1 tbsp garlic-infused oil
1 tbsp dried parsley
1 tbsp freshly chopped parsley

---

1. Add the pepper and rice to the slow cooker and stir.
2. Stir in the chopped tomatoes with 2 cups of boiling water.
3. Add in the heated fish stock, cover, then cook on Low for 2 hours.
4. Uncover, then stir – the rice should have soaked up most of the liquid.
5. Stir in the mussels, garlic oil, and dried parsley.
6. (Hint: You can add a splash more water if the rice is looking dry.)
7. Cook for 10 minutes or until the mussels are cooked through.
8. Sprinkle with fresh parsley to serve in large bowls.

Hint: make sure to discard any mussels in the shell that don't open during or after cooking.

Per serving: Calories: 405 Protein: 20g Carbs: 58g Fiber: 3g Sugar: 5g Fat: 11g
(Unsaturated: 8g Saturated: 2g)

Shrimp in Sweet and Sour Broth

SERVES 2 / PREP TIME: 10 MINUTES / COOK TIME: 40 MINUTES LOW + 10 MINUTES

These distinctive sweet and sour flavors complement the shrimp well.

---

3 tbsp rice vinegar or white wine vinegar

2 cups low FODMAP chicken stock

1 tbsp gluten free soy sauce

1 tbsp maple syrup

1 tsp ground ginger

3 green onions (green tips only), thinly sliced

½ cup canned pineapple, diced and juices drained

6 oz small raw peeled shrimp

---

1. Add the vinegar, stock, soy sauce, syrup and ginger to the slow cooker.
2. Add the green onions and cook on Low for 40 minutes
3. The sauce should have thickened by this point.
4. Add in the pineapple and heat through for 10 minutes.
5. Add the shrimp for 5 minutes or until thoroughly cooked through.

Per serving: Calories: 187 Protein: 21g Carbs: 20g Fiber: 1g Sugar: 12g Fat: 3g (Unsaturated: 2g Saturated: 1g)

Lemon and Cilantro Salmon

SERVES 6 / PREP TIME: 5 MINUTES / COOK TIME: 1 1/2 HOURS HIGH

Zesty and juicy salmon on a bed of soft rice.

1 lb salmon fillet, cut into 4 meal size
portions
A pinch of salt and pepper
2 lemons, juice
2 tbsp fresh cilantro, finely chopped
½ cup cooked green beans to serve
1 cup cooked white rice

1. Line a piece of parchment paper into the slow cooker base.
2. Place the 4 salmon fillets flat on the parchment paper.
3. Sprinkle each with a little salt and pepper over the top.
4. Drizzle lemon juice over the salmon pieces and sprinkle with chopped cilantro.
5. Set on High and cook for 1 hour or 1 ½ hours for thicker cuts.
6. Once salmon is cooked, carefully lift out of the slow cooker.
7. Place into a shallow serving dish.
8. Remove the skin and serve.
9. Plate up with green beans and rice.

Per serving: Calories: 153 Protein: 20g Carbs: 10g Fiber: 1g Sugar: 1g Fat: 3g
(Unsaturated: 2g Saturated: 1g)

Slow-Cooked Calamari

SERVES 4 / PREP TIME: 5 MINUTES / COOK TIME: 20 MINUTES LOW

Calamari is rich in copper and selenium – two essential vitamins that work as antioxidants in your body. This serving alone contains more than your daily requirement of copper – great if you're lacking on other days!

---

8 oz raw calamari
1 medium yellow pepper, diced
1 ½ large red peppers, diced
1 cup green beans
1 tbsp coconut oil
1 tbsp freshly chopped parsley
1 cup water
1 tsp salt

---

1. Add all ingredients to a slow cooker , stir and cook on Low for 20-25 minutes or until calamari is cooked through but not over done.
2. Serve hot!

Hint: Take care not to over eat calamari, as it is also high in sodium – everything in moderation!

Per serving: Calories: 111 Protein: 10g Carbs: 8g Fiber: 2g Sugar:2g Fat: 5g (Unsaturated: 2g Saturated: 3g)

Seafood Bisque

SERVES 6 / PREP TIME: 5 MINUTES / COOK TIME: 4 HOURS LOW + 1 HOUR

A tasty mix of seafood with a herby sauce.

1 ½ cups chopped beef tomatoes
2 cups low FODMAP chicken/fish stock
2 celery stalks, finely sliced
1 medium red bell pepper, finely chopped
1 tsp dried thyme
8 oz crab meat, fresh or frozen
7 oz large size raw shrimp, rinsed

1. Tip in the tomatoes, stock and vegetables to the slow cooker.
2. Add the thyme and cook for 4 hours on Low.
3. (Hint: If you're in a rush, cook for 2 hours on High.)
4. Add the crab meat and shrimp and cook for another hour on Low.
5. Remove from the heat and serve.

Per serving: Calories: 123 Protein: 18g Carbs: 6g Fiber: 1g Sugar: 3g Fat: 2g
(Unsaturated: 2g Saturated: 0g)

Shrimp and Yellow Pepper Jambalaya

SERVES 6 / PREP TIME: 10 MINUTES / COOK TIME: 7 HOURS + 1 HOUR LOW

A vibrant and tasty dish.

---

1 lb uncooked peeled shrimp
4 cups cooked brown rice
28 oz diced beef tomatoes
1 cup chopped yellow bell pepper
1 tbsp parsley
1 cup chopped celery stalks
¼ tsp ground black pepper
½ tsp chopped chives
½ tsp sea salt

---

1. Hold the shrimp and rice to one side.
2. Place all the other ingredients into a slow cooker.
3. Cover and cook for 7 hours on Low. Add in the shrimp, rice and 8 cups water.
4. Cover and cook for another hour on Low.
5. Alternatively cook on High for 4 hours and then add the shrimp for 30 minutes on High.
6. Serve hot.

Per serving: Calories: 184 Protein: 14g Carbs: 27g Fiber: 4g Sugar: 7g Fat: 2g (Unsaturated: 2g Saturated: 0g)

Thai Clams with Rice

SERVES 8 / PREP TIME: 5 MINUTES / COOK TIME: 4 HOURS + 50 MINUTES LOW

A delicious Thai infused clam dish with ginger and lime.

---

2 medium yellow bell peppers, sliced
1 ½ cups rice
10 slices of grated fresh ginger peeled
32 oz low FODMAP fish stock
14 oz almond milk
¼ cup sliced green onions (green tips only)

2 cups fresh green beans, ends trimmed
15 oz fresh clams
1/3 cup fresh lime juice

---

1. Place the bell peppers, rice, and ginger into the slow cooker.
2. Pour in the fish stock and milk.
3. Stir well, cover and cook for 4 hours on Low or 2 hours on High.
4. Add the green onions and green beans.
5. Stir in the clams and lime juice.
6. Cover and cook for another 50 minutes on Low.
7. Transfer into serving bowls and enjoy.

Per serving: Calories: 164 Protein: 6g Carbs: 31g Fiber: 1g Sugar: 4g Fat: 2g (Unsaturated: 1g Saturated: 0g)

DRINKS AND DESSERTS

Quick-Blitzed Banana Smoothie

SERVES 1 / PREP TIME: 5 MINUTES / COOK TIME: NA

Cold, refreshing and nutritious.

1/2 banana, peeled and sliced
½ cup almond milk
Handful of ice
1 tbsp maple syrup (optional)
1/2 tsp ground nutmeg

---

1. Place all of the ingredients into a blender.
2. Blitz until smooth.
3. Transfer to a serving glass and serve at once.

Per serving: Calories: 157 Protein: 1g Carbs: 35g Fiber: 2g Sugar: 29g Fat: 2g
(Unsaturated: 2g Saturated: 0g)

Raspberry and Cranberry Juice Blend

SERVES 2 / PREP TIME: 5 MINUTES / COOK TIME: NA

Deliciously refreshing.

---

1 cup cranberry juice
½ cup frozen organic raspberries, defrosted
Cup rice milk
1 tbsp brown sugar, or to taste
2 mint sprigs, to serve

---

1. Place all the ingredients into a blender and pulse until smooth.
2. Pour into glasses and serve topped with fresh mint.

Per serving: Calories: 156 Protein: 4g Carbs: 32g Fiber: 4g Sugar: 25g Fat: 2g (Unsaturated: 2g Saturated: 0g)

Blueberry Pancake Shake

SERVES 2 / PREP TIME: 5 MINUTES / COOK TIME: NA

Sweet and delicious - a real treat.

½ cup organic blueberries
1 tbsp maple syrup
1 tsp vanilla extract
1 cup almond milk

---

1. In a blender, add all the ingredients and blitz them up.
2. Pour into milkshake glasses and enjoy.

Per serving: Calories: 100 Protein: 1g Carbs: 20g Fiber: 1g Sugar: 18g Fat: 1g (Unsaturated: 1g Saturated: 0g)

Classic Strawberry Shake

SERVES 1 / PREP TIME: 5 MINUTES / COOK TIME: NA

Perfect to satisfy any milkshake cravings.

1/2 cup crushed ice
½ cup rice milk
1/2 banana, peeled and sliced
3 strawberries, halved
Handful of organic strawberries, plus
extra to garnish

---

1. Add ice to blender and pulse until you get fine pieces.
2. While ice is being crushed, measure the rice milk.
3. Add the milk and fruit and blend for approximately 1 minute or until smooth.
4. Serve.

Per serving: Calories: 132 Protein: 2g Carbs: 30gg Fiber: 4g Sugar: 20g Fat: 2g
(Unsaturated: 1g Saturated: 0g)

Rhubarb and Strawberry Crumble

SERVES 6 / PREP TIME: 10 MINUTES / COOK TIME: 2 1/2 HOURS HIGH

Fantastically tart and sweet with crumbly oaty topping.

---

3 cups organic strawberries, sliced
3 cups rhubarb, sliced
½ cup sugar
1 tbsp lemon zest
1 cup gluten free oats
¼ tsp ground nutmeg
½ cup very ripe banana, mashed

---

1. In a slow cooker, toss together the strawberries, rhubarb, sugar and lemon zest.
2. In a medium bowl, stir together the oats and nutmeg.
3. Mix in the mashed banana with your fingertips, crumbling until large 'breadcrumbs' are formed.
4. Heap this on top of the strawberry and rhubarb mixture.
5. Cover and cook on High for 2 ½ hours or until fruit is bubbling
6. Your topping will be crisp and lightly golden brown.
7. Spoon into bowls and enjoy.

Per serving: Calories: 178 Protein: 3g Carbs: 43g Fiber: 6g Sugar: 24g Fat: 1g
(Unsaturated: 0g Saturated: 0g)

Tropical Fruit Crumble

SERVES 6 / PREP TIME: `0 MINUTES / COOK TIME: 2 1/2 HOURS HIGH

Classic crumble with an exotic twist.

---

1 tsp olive oil
3 cups sliced mandarin, orange and pineapple
3 nectarines, sliced
¼ cup sugar
2 tbsp rice flour
1 tsp grated lemon peel
2 tbsp brown sugar
¼ tsp ground nutmeg
¼ cup very ripe banana, mashed

---

1. Lightly oil the bottom of your slow cooker.
2. Add the mandarin, nectarines, sugar, rice flour and lemon peel, and toss them together.
3. In a medium bowl, mix the brown sugar, nutmeg, and banana.
4. Cut in the banana with a pastry blender or by criss-crossing two knives until the mixture looks like coarse sand.
5. You should be able to pinch the mixture and have it hold its shape.
6. Scatter the mixture over the top of the fruit.
7. Cover and cook on High for 2½ hours until the fruit is bubbling.
8. Spoon into bowls and serve hot.

Per serving: Calories: 127 Protein: 2g Carbs: 31g Fiber: 3g Sugar: 25g Fat: 0g (Unsaturated: 0g Saturated: 0g)

Creamy Rice Pudding

SERVES 8 / PREP TIME: 10 MINUTES / COOK TIME: 3 HOURS LOW

A family favorite - warming and sweet.

3 cups cooked dessert rice
8 tbsp raisins
1 tsp vanilla extract
1 ½ cups coconut milk
1 tbsp sugar
1 tsp ground cinnamon

1. Line your slow cooker with a little coconut oil.
2. Mix all the ingredients except sugar and cinnamon in the slow cooker.
3. Cover and cook on Low for 3 hours.
4. The liquid should be absorbed by this point.
5. Stir the pudding.
6. Sprinkle with the sugar and the cinnamon to finish.
7. Serve warm.

Per serving: Calories: 216 Protein:3g Carbs: 28g Fiber: 2g Sugar: 9g Fat: 11g
(Unsaturated:1g Saturated: 10g)

CONVERSION TABLES

Volume

Imperial	Metric
1 tbsp	15ml
2 fl oz	55 ml
3 fl oz	75 ml
5 fl oz (¼ pint)	150 ml
10 fl oz (½ pint)	275 ml
1 pint	570 ml
1 ¼ pints	725 ml
1 ¾ pints	1 liter
2 pints	1.2 liters
2½ pints	1.5 liters
4 pints	2.25 liters

Oven temperatures

Gas Mark	Fahrenheit	Celsius
1/4	225	110
1/2	250	130
1	275	140
2	300	150
3	325	170
4	350	180
5	375	190
6	400	200
7	425	220
8	450	230
9	475	240

Weight

Imperial	Metric
½ oz	10 g
¾ oz	20 g
1 oz	25 g
1½ oz	40 g
2 oz	50 g
2½ oz	60 g
3 oz	75 g
4 oz	110 g
4½ oz	125 g
5 oz	150 g
6 oz	175 g
7 oz	200 g
8 oz	225 g
9 oz	250 g
10 oz	275 g
12 oz	350 g

BIBLIOGRAPHY

FODMAP food list (2017) Available at: http://www.ibsdiets.org/FODMAP-diet/FODMAP-food-list/ (Accessed: 22 February 2017).

Micawber (no date) Dangers of avoidance. Available at: http://www.ibs-health.com/page284.html (Accessed: 22 February 2017).

Ross, E. and Lam, M. (2016) 'The low FODMAPS diet and IBS: A winning strategy', Journal of Clinical Nutrition and Dietetics, 02(01). doi: 10.4172/2472-1921.100013.

Camilleri, M. and Acosta, A. (2014) 'Re: Halmos et al, A diet low in FODMAPs reduces symptoms of irritable bowel syndrome', Gastroenterology, 146(7), pp. 1829–1830. doi: 10.1053/j.gastro.2014.01.071.

Gibson, P.R., Varney, J.E. and Muir, J.G. (2016) 'Diet therapy for irritable bowel syndrome: Is a diet low in FODMAPS really similar in efficacy to traditional dietary advice?', Gastroenterology, 150(4), pp. 1046–1047. doi: 10.1053/j.gastro.2015.10.053.

Piacentino, D., Rossi, S., Piretta, L., Badiali, D., Pallotta, N. and Corazziari, E. (2016) 'Tu1425 role of FODMAPs, and benefit of Low-FODMAP diet, in irritable bowel syndrome severity', Gastroenterology, 150(4), p. S901. doi: 10.1016/s0016-5085(16)33048-7.

Chung, C.-Y. and Joo, Y.-E. (2014) 'Can a diet low in Fermentable Oligosaccharides, Disaccharides, Monosaccharides and polyols (FODMAPs) reduce the symptoms of irritable bowel syndrome?', The Korean Journal of Gastroenterology, 64(2), p. 123. doi: 10.4166/kjg.2014.64.2.123.

BS: Risk of IBS increases after bacterial infection (2015) Nature Reviews Gastroenterology and Hepatology, 12(6), pp. 313–313. doi: 10.1038/nrgastro.2015.86.

Sidebar (1998) Available at: http://www.aboutibs.org (Accessed: 23 February 2017).

INDEX